W0234983

"*The Somato-Psychic Realm: Analytic Receptivity and Resonance* is an extraordinary collection of essays exploring the interplay between the somatic and psychic realms in psychoanalytic theory and practice. Each chapter, written by distinguished scholars and clinicians, carefully examines Bion's revolutionary concepts and their influence on contemporary psychoanalysis. Rich with clinical illustrations emphasizing the inseparability of mind and body, this volume is essential for psychoanalysts and scholars wishing to deepen their understanding of Bion's legacy and the development of analytic thought."

Giuseppe Civitarese, *author of* On Arrogance: A Psychoanalytic Essay,
London 2023

"In a brilliant contribution to psychoanalysis the editors extend its reach to the non-sensuous realm of the unrepresented, demystifying and exploring what Bion called O. Since language fails to reach this undifferentiated proto-mental level of functioning, the analyst must meet the patient by using his somatic registrations, 'feeling in (his) flesh.' Nine international analysts contribute chapters elucidating the clinical challenges and opportunities of working at this deepest level: offering a vitalizing presence and availability to the patient requires an expanded use of oneself."

Karen Roos, *Boston Psychoanalytic Institute and Society, USA*

"Like shafts of light in the darkness, this book offers pioneering contemporary insight into the most vital dimension of psychoanalysis today, where both pathos and mutative change are found in the shared, inchoate movements of embodied life. From different but related perspectives, ten eminent scholars of the nameless regions charted by Freud, Winnicott, and Bion show how analysts are captured by and work with unintegrated traumatic experiences that change them as it does their patients by giving the inexpressible some form. Dolan and David Power have crafted an indispensable guide for all who traverse this challenging but transformative domain."

Jack Foehl, *Joint Editor in Chief*, Psychoanalytic Dialogues, Past President, Boston Psychoanalytic Society and Institute

The Somato-Psychic Realm

Influenced by the groundbreaking work of Wilfred Bion, *The Somato-Psychic Realm: Analytic Receptivity and Resonance* sees ten internationally acclaimed psychoanalysts explore the complex interrelationship between our psychic and somatic selves, and highlight its promising riches and devastating disruptions.

Explored theoretically and illustrated with vivid clinical examples, the contributors in this volume map our current understanding on the fascinating subject of psychic and somatic selves, reframing it as the 'somato-psychic realm'. This collection of essays brings together the current thinking, reflections, and clinical understanding of prominent Bionian psychoanalytic practitioners and scholars, from Rudi Vermote to Judy Eekhoff, each of whom have developed particular interests and expertise in analytically approaching the realm of the somato-psychic. The reader is offered extensions of theory and vivid clinical examples and invited to consider many questions central to contemporary psychoanalytic practice: does the body think and if so, how does the analyst converse with it? Is thinking in a psychoanalytic sense best conceived of as a combined function of the soma and psyche? How does this perspective reorient analytic technique? Can we conceptualize a body-to-body dimension of the analytic experience, and in the analytic encounter how does this dimension serve a vitalizing function for the patient while remaining outside of the usual verbal and symbolizing exchanges between analyst and patient? What is the fate of failures and disruptions in the somato-psychic interrelationship and how does the analyst hear, recognize, and respond to these failures? How does the analyst make subjective space to experience in herself the presence of these disruptions? What transformations in our technical stance does this type of clinical presentation require? As they approach the challenges of the somato-psychic realm, readers will find themselves drawn into this conversation, invited by a thought-provoking foreword by Patrick Miller.

It will be a vital resource for psychoanalysts in training and practice alike looking for a greater recognition of and ability to respond to problems ranging from frank somatic disorders to failures in symbolization and thought process and the non-neurotic states of mind that accompany these disorders.

David G. Power is a founding member of The Boston Group for Psychoanalytic Studies (BGPS), a past President, Supervisory and Teaching Analyst at the Massachusetts Institute for Psychoanalysis and on the faculty of the Boston Psychoanalytic Society and Institute. With Howard Levine, he co-edited *Engaging Primitive Anxieties of the Emerging Self* (2017). He maintains a private practice in psychoanalysis, psychotherapy and supervision in Cambridge, Massachusetts.

Dolan Power is a founding member of The Boston Group for Psychoanalytic Studies, Past President, Supervisory and Teaching Analyst at the Massachusetts Institute for Psychoanalysis and on the faculty of the Boston Psychoanalytic Society and Institute. She was awarded the Francis Tustin Memorial Prize in 2011 for her paper "The Use of the Analyst as an Autistic Shape" (IJP 2016). She maintains a private practice in psychoanalysis, consultation and supervision in Cambridge, Massachusetts.

The Somato-Psychic Realm

Analytic Receptivity and Resonance

Edited by
David G. Power and Dolan Power
Foreword by Patrick Miller

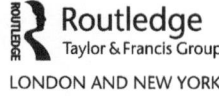
Routledge
Taylor & Francis Group

LONDON AND NEW YORK

Designed cover image: Getty Images. Vertigo 3D

First published 2025
by Routledge
4 Park Square, Milton Park, Abingdon, Oxon OX14 4RN

and by Routledge
605 Third Avenue, New York, NY 10158

Routledge is an imprint of the Taylor & Francis Group, an informa business

© 2025 selection and editorial matter, David G. Power and Dolan Power; individual chapters, the contributors

The right of David G. Power and Dolan Power to be identified as the authors of the editorial material, and of the authors for their individual chapters, has been asserted in accordance with sections 77 and 78 of the Copyright, Designs and Patents Act 1988.

All rights reserved. No part of this book may be reprinted or reproduced or utilised in any form or by any electronic, mechanical, or other means, now known or hereafter invented, including photocopying and recording, or in any information storage or retrieval system, without permission in writing from the publishers.

Trademark notice: Product or corporate names may be trademarks or registered trademarks, and are used only for identification and explanation without intent to infringe.

British Library Cataloguing-in-Publication Data
A catalogue record for this book is available from the British Library

ISBN: 978-1-032-87767-9 (hbk)
ISBN: 978-1-032-86443-3 (pbk)
ISBN: 978-1-003-53436-5 (ebk)

DOI: 10.4324/9781003534365

Typeset in Times New Roman
by Taylor & Francis Books

Contents

This book is dedicated to our patients, from whom we have learned so much over the years, and to our colleagues and friends who have inspired us, challenged us, taught us, and learned with us through their participation in conferences and clinical seminars sponsored by The Boston Group for Psychoanalytic Studies.

Contributors

João Carlos Braga graduated in Medicine from the Federal University of Paraná, Brazil (1966). He was a fellow at Baylor University, Department of Psychiatry, Houston, Texas (1967). He is a full member, faculty, training and supervising analyst at the Brazilian Psychoanalytic Society of São Paulo and Curitiba's Psychoanalytic Society. He has authored 30 psychoanalytical papers and book chapters published in national and international reviews.

Judy K. Eekhoff is a full faculty member of Northwestern Psychoanalytic Society & Institute and Seattle Psychoanalytic Society & Institute. She is the author of *Trauma and Primitive Mental States: An Object Relations Perspective* and *Bion and Primitive Mental States: Trauma and the Symbiotic Link*. Her third book, *Bion's Emotional Links: Love, Hate, and Knowledge,* is forthcoming from Routledge.

Ofra Eshel is faculty, training and supervising analyst, The Israel Psychoanalytic Society and Institute, honorary member, NCP, Los Angeles, and Founder and Head of the post-graduate track "Independent Psychoanalysis: Radical Breakthroughs" at the advanced studies of the Program of Psychoanalytic Psychotherapy, Faculty of Medicine, Tel-Aviv University. Published widely in many languages, she co-edited *Was It or Was It Not? When Shadows of Sexual Abuse Emerge in Psychoanalytic Treatment* (2017) and authored *The Emergence of Analytic Oneness: Into the Heart of Psychoanalysis* (Routledge, 2019).

Béatrice Ithier is member of the Société psychanalytique de Paris and is recognized as child, adolescent, and adult psychoanalyst by the IPA. She is a full member of the Italian Psychoanalytical Society, Pavia, dual member; a training member of the Warsaw Institute of Psychoanalysis and Psychotherapy; and a member of the European Society of Psychoanalysis (infant and adolescent). Widely published in France and abroad, she edited *En séance au fil de l'affect et de l'émotion, Approches contemporaines,* Paris, Ithaque.

Celia Fix Korbivcher is training, supervising, and child analyst, Brazilia Psychoanalytic Society of São Paulo. Her papers have appeared in Brazilian and international journals, including the *IJP*. Her book *Autistic Transformations* was published in Portuguese (Imago Ed, 2010), English (Karnac, 2013), and Korean (Instituto de Psicoterapia da Corea, 2015). She received the First International Parthenope Thalamo Bion Prize (2004) and the 9th Frances Tustin Memorial Prize (2005).

Howard B. Levine is a member of PINE, the Contemporary Freudian Society, Pulsion, and NYU Postdoc's Contemporary Freudian Track. He is on the Editorial Board of the IJP and Psychoanalytic Inquiry, Editor-in-Chief of the *Routledge Wilfred Bion Studies Book Series*, and in private practice in Brookline, Massachusetts. He is the editor or co-editor of many books and is the author of *Transformations de l'Irreprésentable* (Ithaque, 2019) and *Affect, Representation and Language: Between the Silence and the Cry* (Routledge, 2022).

Patrick Miller trained in Paris, studying with Piera Aulagnier and Andre Green. He co-founded the Societe Psychanalytique de Recherche et de Formation in Paris in 2005, serving as president from 2007–2011. An IPA training analyst and member of CAPS in Princeton, he has authored numerous papers in international journals, and published two books, *Le Psychanalyste pendant la Séance* (2001) and *Driving Soma: A Transformational Process in the Analytic Encounter* (2014). He practices in Paris.

Bernd Nissen is a psychoanalyst (DPV/IPA) in private practice in Berlin, Germany. His areas of interest include metapsychological, theoretical, and clinical conceptualization of autistoid and nameless states, and reflections on "time" and "space" in psychic systems. He is the Co-editor of the Yearbook of Psychoanalysis. His publications appear in numerous languages.

David G. Power is a founding member of The Boston Group for Psychoanalytic Studies (BGPS), a past President, Supervisory and Teaching Analyst at the Massachusetts Institute for Psychoanalysis, and on the faculty of the Boston Psychoanalytic Society and Institute. He co-edited with Howard Levine *Engaging Primitive Anxieties of the Emerging Self* (Karnac, 2017). He practices in Cambridge, Massachusetts.

Dolan Power is a founding member of The Boston Group for Psychoanalytic Studies, Past President, Supervisory and Teaching Analyst at the Massachusetts Institute for Psychoanalysis, and on the Faculty of the Boston Psychoanalytic Society and Institute. She was awarded the Francis Tustin Memorial Prize in 2011 for her paper "The Use of the Analyst as an Autistic Shape" (*IJP*, 2016). She maintains a private practice in psychoanalysis, consultation, and supervision in Cambridge, Massachusetts.

Rudi Vermote is training analyst, past president of the Belgian Society of Psychoanalysis, and Professor at the University of Leuven. He has published and lectured on Bion's work and is the author of *Reading Bion* (Routledge, 2019). He is a member of the editorial board of the *IJP* and Honorary Member of the Psychoanalytic Center of California.

Foreword: Unbounded maps, unchartered territories

Patrick Miller

Le silence éternel de ces espaces infinis m'effraie. [The eternal silence of these infinite spaces terrifies me].

(Pascal, 1670/1958, p. 61)

The authors of this book are grappling with the limits of understanding and knowledge in psychoanalytic theory and practice, hence with psychoanalytic tradition. They are the descendants of a lineage that began with Ferenczi and runs through to Winnicott and, above all, Bion. They all testify, each in their own way, of how transformative their encounter with Bion's thinking has been, how they continue to deepen their understanding of his key concepts in their daily encounter with the enigmas posed by traumatic primitive mental states, with a relentless question: how can we manage to break through to the unattainable?

If the expression "the frontier spirit" was not so laden with political innuendos, I could have chosen it as title of my foreword. Gaining territory on the unknown wilderness, relying on one's own inner spirit to push the limit further and making progress by counting on one's own resources. Confronting oneself with the naked truth.[1] In French we say: "culture is what remains, when everything else has been forgotten". Including Bion.

Matter that knows itself

This conquering spirit is very much in line with Freud's. However, our authors' conquest is more akin to the oceanic feeling, which Freud referred to very early states of being one with another (At-one-ment in Bionian language) and said that he had never experienced it personally. Trying to break through the epistemological barrier[2] that keeps us out of the unrepressed unconscious and of the Id, to remain within Freudian concepts, implies a self-transformation within the act of analyzing, which requires a kind of self-oblivion and self-mourning. It also brings one, necessarily, to develop a thinking of the body, of the mind as part of the body, of the soma as different of the already libidinal body-ego, and to ask the question: is the body as soma reachable by the analytic interaction?

Blaise Pascal saw man as caught between two abysses, incapable of seeing the nothing he came from and the infinite that swallows him up: "the *being* that we do have cuts us off from knowledge of first beginnings, which arise out of the *nothing*; and the smallness of our *being* conceals from us the sight of the *infinite*" (Pascal, 1670/1958, p. 19).

The title of Howard Levine's chapter introduces us to one of the main themes in this book: to feel in the flesh as a means of reaching a co-created meaningful experience in the analytic dyad. If we go one step further, what do we make of the question: to feel *with* the flesh? A question that 17th-century Pascal, who didn't like Descartes, pushes even further: "there being nothing so inconceivable as to say that matter knows itself. It is impossible to imagine how it should know itself" (Pascal, 1670/1958, p. 21).

Although not stated as such, it is a question that arises from several of the chapters. What is the self-knowledge of living matter, if any, and how is it conveyed in the subject's experience of themselves and through what channels can it be conveyed to another and transformed into elements that can be metabolized by the mind?

In the same vein, Judy Eekhoff says that unconscious to unconscious reception can occur through resonances in the body of the analyst, which I understand as the libidinal body of the analyst. However, she goes one step further when she writes: "these impressions present as **somatic** counter-transference" (Eekhoff, Chapter 9, p. 131, my italics).

If I understand well, it means, in Bionian terms, that Beta elements are taken up in the countertransference without having been transformed by the alpha function of the reverie, but can, nonetheless, contribute to the analytic process as such.

I think that we find a similar idea in Celia Fix Korbivcher: "unintegrated transformations occur in an unintegrated medium. They can be identified by the presence of intense unmentalized corporeal manifestations" (Korbivcher, see note 3, Chapter 8, p. 126).

Bernd Nissen invites us to circle the nameless while Mrs. A uses words to describe abhorrent things she does that do not evoke anything in him,[3] leave him feelingless. He points to "a moment of presence" when at last he can have a taste of what the patient experiences and draws on what he senses to be able to tell her this terrible sentence: "This is how you are going to die". The nameless ends up being felt and named.[4]

Since brass, nor stone, nor earth, nor boundless sea,

But sad mortality o'ersways their power.

(Shakespeare, n.d.)

The finite and the infinite are recurring themes in Bion's thinking. There is no end to the potentialities of free-association, or of a session, or of a dream, connecting us, through its navel, as Freud stated in 1900, to the unknown.

An attempt to further Bion's thinking eventually brings his followers to explore the body-mind issue, or rather to confront themselves with the following question: is the barrier impenetrable between psychic life and somatic life?

Rudi Vermote invites the reader to plunge into the infinity of the soma, as a kind of abysmal reflection of the frightening infinite of outer space:

> there are some hundred trillion existing neural connections in the human brain ... 1000 times more than the number of stars in our galaxy ... our microbiome has 39 trillion cells ... is it possible to talk about the infinite body with some poor concepts of psychoanalysis...?
>
> (Chapter 5, p. 71)

To the "poor concepts" Vermote adds what he calls "the wall of language", emphasizing the limitations of verbal thinking and calls to "de-structure language" in order to make contact with the soma possible. However, one might argue that language is deeply rooted in the soma and not simply an abstract super-structure. From this biological dimension of language, we could also turn to poetry where the poesies of the act of speech brings the non-existent into being. In the talking cure, when it is relying on free association combined with the self-hypnotic state induced in the analyst by evenly-floating attention,[5] is language restrictive in itself, or is it a use of language dissociated from the body that creates a limitation?

Piera Aulagnier (1975/2001) believed that psyche borrows from the soma for its shaping and construction. As usual it is quite difficult to describe how the psyche evolves from and out of the soma in a monistic way and not in a dualistic way of thinking. The use of "borrows" is quite meaningful but it implicitly induces the notion of a pre-existing psyche. We find this aporia expressed in its most condensed way by Freud as he was dying: "psyche is extended. Doesn't know about it" (Freud, 1941, p. 300).

I believe that the proximity of death, the impending return to the extension of matter, had a lot to do with the way in which Freud shaped his thought in language.

In the same creative vein as Vermote, biologist Wolf Hervé Fridman wrote in his book *The Mobile Brain, From immunity to the immune system* (1991, p. 47):

> The molecules that make up the immune system, antibodies in particular, possess images of the universe within themselves ... Where is this immunological brain? Everywhere and everywhere at the same time ... The cells that make it up circulate constantly throughout the organism, taking in information, digesting it, communicating it to other cells, multiplying

and taking action. A mobile brain, constantly enriched with new cells, constantly awake, is present in every part of our body.

The representations in the molecules that Fridman talks about exist in a different state of matter than the mental representations in the psyche, and I don't conceive of a linear causality that would run from one to the other. I'm simply taking up a notion: that of borrowing from the somatic in order to model the psychic, with this question: to what extent, in the infinitely small world of somatic operating mechanisms, can we imagine possible borrowings for psychic organization? And, in turn, can we think that the quality of the borrowing may have a decisive impact on the psyche's capacity to influence the soma, hence another way of looking at dissociative states of being between psyche and soma.

Regression or transformation into O?

Judy Eekhoff explores primitive mental states where severe early trauma results in "a primal dissociation of severing the body mind union" and the defense is by using the body and the senses, via a "defensive foregrounding of sensation" (Chapter 9, p. 130). One wonders what can be called "mind" in those early states of being and Eekhoff emphasizes that those are unmentalized and unrepresented mental states. Are they totally unrepresented, or unrepresented in terms of psyche? We fall back on Pascal's question: matter that knows itself.

She addresses the question of regression first through the capacity for projective identification in both analysand and analyst. When those processes are damaged, the analyst is compelled to find another way of establishing contact with the sequestered unmentalized areas in the analysand's being. The world the analyst must try to enter "is a world of body relations, of synchrony and rhythmicity, of sound and sensation. It is a world of music and dance. It is a mysterious world outside the symbolic order" (p. 132).

I would say that in her Bionian perspective, the necessity for formal regression seems to be more on the analyst's side, enabling her to implement the "discipline" of no memory, no desire and reach a state of hallucinosis. However, I am not even sure that this Bionian perspective needs the metapsychological notion of formal regression. It seems that what happens (or doesn't happen) in the state of no memory, no desire, has more to do with a kind of *shift* rather than with a regression. How this shift happens is not clearly theorized but it seems to be deeply related to whether the analyst needs to defend her/his narcissism or is able to suspend it and enter a state of selflessness with a transpersonal dimension.

Hence the importance of quoting Bion himself on this topic of regression:

Winnicott says patients *need* to regress: Melanie Klein says they *must* not: I say they *are* regressed, and the regression should be observed and interpreted by the analyst without any need to compel the patient to become totally regressed before he can make the analyst observe and interpret the regression.

(Bion, 1992, p. 166, italics in original)

This is quite an important point, on which, I believe, not all ten authors would agree. Those who are equally inspired by Winnicott would tend to insist on the necessity for the patient to regress to primary dependence. Are the two positions compatible at different moments of the cure, is a question that could be addressed.

However, Judy Eekhoff points out a possible *defensive use of regression* to symbiosis, not compatible, if I understand her well, with a commensal use of the container/contained interaction because "undifferentiation between self and object wipes out an object to project into" (p. 134). In Winnicottian terms one could argue that experiencing, in the here and now through regression to undifferentiation, the creative illusion of omnipotence creates the opportunity of a new beginning into "being".

The theme of "being" is taken up by Ofra Eshel,[6] described on the analyst's side of the experience, allowing a "being O" rather than knowing O. She quotes Bion:

In so far as the analyst becomes O, he is able to know the events that are the *evolutions* of O. Restating this in terms of psycho-analytic experience, the psychoanalyst can know what the patient says, does, and appears to be, but cannot know the O of which the patient is an evolution: he can only "be" it.

(Bion, 1970, p. 27, italics in original)

In this imagined dialogue, pursuing the defensive use of symbiosis, Eekhoff underlines the necessity of taking a slightly more active stance, calling the patient forth, because "when patients have withdrawn so far into themselves or exploded into infinite space, it is very hard to be with them. It is difficult to be open and receptive to the nothingness of mindless states".

Alvarez said: "Hey, there!", Eekhoff says "Come, come". A bit of doing, for the sake of being. As a result of her attempts to find her patient Dennis, someday, some years down the road, he says: "I felt solid, like I have an inside. I walked around the house saying, I'm alive, I'm alive" (Chapter 9, p. 138).

A breath of life

When, after 1920, Freud needed to conceptualize a new topography, he replaced the System Ucs by a less clear-cut region described as a reservoir of drives, a chaos, a seething cauldron, the dark, inaccessible part of our personality. His first drawing, or diagram, is of a horizontal form, showing an encapsulated region called ID (Freud, 1923, p. 24). Ten years later, his drawing is vertical and the ID region is wide open into the soma. He writes that different areas of the mind are best represented, not by a drawing "but rather by areas of colour melting into one another as they are presented by modern artists" (Freud, 1933[1932], p. 79).

Freud borrowed the term Id, from Groddeck's It (1923/1979), and conceptualized it in quite a different way. However, one may remember that Groddeck tied the notion of It to the most elemental forms of life. For him, the It begins with fertilization and ends with the life of an individual, although, he thinks, the moment at which we can say an individual is dead is not a simple matter.

The It is a powerful life force which pervades the individual unless it is hindered and turns into disease:

> I hold the view that man is animated by the Unknown, that there is within him an "Es," an "It," some wondrous force which directs both what he himself does, and what happens to him. The affirmation "I live" is only conditionally correct, it expresses only a small and superficial part of the fundamental principle, "Man is lived by the It".
>
> (Groddeck 1923/1979, p. 9)

I find an echo of Groddeck's It in Dolan Power's representation of the proto-mental as "a background state of being that remains undifferentiated, elemental to being alive" (Chapter 1, p. 12). She reminds us that "Bion's emphasis was always on movement, circularity, porosity, and permeability, rather than anchoring the concept in a particular bodily or sensory experience" (p. 11). She also stresses two very important differences.

The proto-mental being a continuous experience throughout life, as a "foundational state of being" should not be confused with primitive mental states. Actually, although in a very different metapsychological perspective, I find the notion of the proto-mental, as seen in that dimension, quite close to what Piera Aulagnier (1975/2001) conceptualized as the "pictographic activity in the original dimension", which remains out of reach as such, is continuous throughout life, and foundational of all capacities for figuration and representation.

Another difference is with the Beta elements. The proto-mental is associated in Bion's mind with an ongoing involuntary flow, best illustrated by breathing or blood circulating through the capillary system, whereas Beta elements, as elements, are defined (i.e not undifferentiated) and arise out of the proto-mental. They "are related to the sensorial experience and are part of the perceptual system" (p. 13).

How does the analyst's own proto-mental experience, as an ongoing state of being, resonate with the patient's, how does it manage to establish a contact or a connection, and how does that capacity of connection and apprehension enable a possibility to re-orient the analysand's proto-mental towards more aliveness when the proto-mental has been maimed by a "nameless dread"? Béatrice Ithier describes a remarkable clinical moment where she utters a sentence, unprepared and uncontrolled, by which she is herself startled, stemming out of an unconscious ongoing process of interpretation, which has managed to find its way to word representations. It (Groddeck) comes out of the analyst's mouth, in a way that is reminiscent of the Pythia of Delphi.

This question goes back to Freud's early interrogations about a direct communication from unconscious to unconscious,[7] even though Freud's unconscious of 1912 is not Bion's proto-mental. But the issue is similar: how does the life of the unknown, of unconscious representations or of the unrepresented capture and convey a meaning in ways, as Freud notes, that are inaccessible to us?

Interrogations about the proto-mental inevitably lead us to the last section of my introduction: how does pre-natal life relate to post-natal life?

Caesura or not Caesura?

In "Observations on transference love", to describe the analytic process, Freud used the parallel of pregnancy, the most bodily and symbolic metaphor of growth and transformation. When Freud in 1926 insisted that there might be more continuity between pre-natal and post-natal life, he used the word "caesura", which was later picked up by Bion.[8]

Celia Fix Korbivcher writes that "[Bion] suggests that the pre-natal sensations could be the origin of proto-emotions, including states of subthalamic terror" (Chapter 8, p. 119).

These "inaccessible states of mind" (Bion, 1975) (but are they states of *mind?*) are not influenced by the mind, do not acquire meaning, and are expressed by somatic manifestations rather than by bodily manifestations. However, they certainly influence the way in which the psychical dimension develops, the quality of the "background state of being" defined as the proto-mental by D. Power.[9]

In my experience as an analyst, some incidents during the process of birth (for instance a sudden interruption of some kind) can, in an après-coup effect, reinforce some patterns of destiny lived as repetition compulsion, giving an excessive momentum to the repetition. For example, a repetitive pattern of events in life and in the transference, that becomes identifiable in the course of an analysis by the patient in the form of "everything starts well, but then irrepressibly turns sour and negative". This repetitive pattern comes to be worked through in the analysis within the dimension of the oedipal organization, the unconscious fantasy life, dreams, unconscious guilt, perhaps negative therapeutic reaction, all different aspects and levels of psychic representability. A lot comes to be worked through and understood at a deep level, allowing for transformations. The repetition compulsion becomes less forceful, but is, nevertheless, still present. In the light of certain affects and emotions linked to sensations that come up in the sessions, representations of a traumatic birth experience may come up in the analyst's mind and eventually be shared with the patient. Then a parental narrative of a traumatic birth may come back to the patient's mind, or the patient may ask his parents about the circumstance of her/his birth. Then this proto-mental experience can become integrated as a thinkable history, the proto-history becoming part of the subject's history, within a complex, non-linear, causality.

In his introduction to *The Trauma of Birth*, Otto Rank raises a question closely linked to those interrogations:

> the deepest biological content ultimately almost unchanged, though indiscernible only through our own inner repression, yet remains tangible as manifest form even in the highest intellectual accomplishments. ... the chief purpose of this work is to draw attention to this *biologically based law of the form which determines the content.*
>
> (Rank, 1929, p. 5, italics in the original)

Rank considered the trauma of birth as a primal organizer of psychic life, a precursor of separation anxiety, death anxiety, and castration anxiety. Having in mind the birth trauma as background, Rank works his way up the whole chain of drive transformations.[10] Lacking space here to go further into Rank's thinking, I can only recommend reading this almost forgotten pioneer of psychoanalysis, who, in 1923, began sketching interrogations, especially around regression and the biologically rooted mind, that contemporary psychoanalysis is still grappling with.

Seen from Rank's perspective, the trauma is the violent ejection out of the mother's womb, and the sudden falling into a completely different environment. The accent is on the caesura as a foundational moment. What happens to the prenatal proto-mental inscriptions, and what the trauma of birth does to them, remains an open-ended question.

At this point I would like to bring in a little detour in the hallucinatory satisfaction of need. What do infants hallucinate, and in what form? At this early stage, it is difficult to think of it as a hallucinatory representation of the object giving the breast or performing some action to relieve a painful tension. The experience of real satisfaction is accompanied by all sorts of bodily sensations, accompanied by affects of pleasure or unpleasure, which act both as a representation of the experience and as a representation of the source object of that experience, an object which, at this stage, is not recognized and represented as separate from the infants' internal states.

From my point of view, the various elements and mechanisms that come into play to form this experience known as the hallucinatory satisfaction of need can be represented as follows. Under the pressure of unpleasant endosomatic tension, and in search of the identity of perception, the infant's organism manages to self-procure the equivalent of the experience of satisfaction, by succeeding in triggering within himself sensations more or less equivalent to those it experiences during the experience of real satisfaction. This set of self-induced somatic sensations allows him to soothe the painful sensation of tension linked to the need, as if the need had been satisfied, even though the need persists in the body. This allows the infant to wait.

This waiting function indicates that this hallucinatory experience is already fulfilling the role that will later be played by the psychic apparatus.

For me, it's important to emphasize that what is self-procured are bodily sensations that reproduce what is experienced in real satisfaction, and not a hallucination as such. It's a moment of becoming psychic of somatic sensation. These sensations have the value of representation (and of a lure corresponding to the identity of perception). The organism's ability to trigger these somatic sensations so that they represent an experience of satisfaction that is not actually taking place is also one of the functions of the psychic apparatus. But it is clear that this first degree of hallucinatory representation involves a hijacking of neuro-physiological functions with the precise aim of calming painful tension in the absence of specific action by the object. This first stage in the development of a hallucinatory capacity, which will form part of the potentialities of psychic life, lies at the boundary between the somatic and the psychic, just like the drive as defined by Freud.

The whole movement that will enable the organism to trigger neurophysiological reactions that will take on the value of representing the experience of satisfaction, prefigures what will become a movement of introjection. This movement, which relies on the body's somatic capacities, could be one of the foundations of the introjection of a maternal capacity. This is the first stage of becoming psychic, contemporary with a potential ability to become autonomous in relation to the object, which is not represented at this stage, but is active in maintaining the illusion of omnipotence (Winnicott) and in its metabolizing function through the alpha function (Bion).

This capacity to trigger somatic sensation into existence may draw on prenatal ways of functioning.

In a recent paper, René Roussillon focuses on a central epistemological issue, with important clinical and technical consequences. The fact that in the first two years of life, the way in which early experiences are recorded is based on processes rather than content, what neuroscientists call "procedural memory", implies a different methodological approach that relies on a special sensitivity to primitive mental states.[11] During fetal life, fundamental needs are met with biological regulation which is not "good enough" but perfect in its total and immediate adaptation to needs:

The foetus receives "everything" it needs, it receives it "straight away" as soon as the need is biologically perceived, it happens "all by itself", it has no effort to make and the biological response is perfectly adapted, it is "at the centre", its needs take precedence over those of its mother, they are satisfied "all the way through."

(Roussillon, 2023, pp. 4–5)

The caesura of birth means a total change of regulation from perfectly adapted biological, to approximately adapted, even if the early maternal preoccupation is very attuned to the infant's needs. Hence the necessity to find in oneself the resources of agency. It is quite likely that the agency (hallucination) relies on the traces left in the organism by the biological regulation, a memory of pre-natal biological regulation, hence bringing it into the psychic construction of the life of the mind.

The first breath is the bodily signifier of a catastrophic change opening up to the possibility of a psychic life thriving on the nostalgia of paradise lost. Psychic elaboration (thinking) versus biological regulation (not yet thinking or thinking in a way totally unknown to us). This may be at the origin of a distinction between Eros and Thanatos, and of the introduction of the death drive, as a powerful wish to not bear the pain of thinking and desiring and to go back to the Nirvana of biological regulation.

Notes

1 Howard Levine: "humans need truth for psychic growth" (Chapter 3, p. 41).
2 W. Bion: "how could we penetrate the caesura of birth?" (quoted by Korbivcher, Chapter 8, p. 120).
3 Words used as a Beta screen?
4 Bernd Nissen: about his other patient, Mrs B.: "This session sounds quite harmless, but it is not. I had never before experienced such naked, nameless horror with such intensity" (Chapter 2, p. 33).
5 "When free-floating attention can be sustained, it has an impact on several dimensions: the relative suspending of the predominance of secondary processes and judgements, putting enactment and reacting on hold, and the capacity to have access to what, in metapsychological terms, we call formal regression. This draws mental functioning in the direction of the hallucinatory dimension and tends to mobilise affects, emotions and feelings. Free-floating attention leads to more bodily availability and permeability" (Miller, 2014, p. 67).
6 "*Thus,* the depths of the unknown, especially the most traumatic unknown, where the patient's emotional reality is mostly unthinkable, unexperienced, and unrepresented, necessitate—by definition—going beyond epistemological exploration to the analytic work of being and becoming with-in the patient's psychic reality, at-one-with the patient's innermost emotional reality. *The unthinkable cannot be thought, but only relived and gone through with or at-one-with the analyst*" (Chapter 6, p. 85, italics in original).
7 "[the analyst] must turn his own unconscious like a receptive organ towards the transmitting unconscious of the patient" (Freud, 1912, p. 115).
8 "There is much more continuity between intra-uterine life and earliest infancy than the impressive caesura of the act of birth would have us believe" (Freud, 1926, p. 138).

9 João Braga: "The somato-psychic realm belongs to Bion's conjectures that the mind has a bedrock—a proto-mental personality—modelled after a prenatal mind that functions independently from the development of postnatal experiences" (Chapter 7, p. 104).
10 "The threat of castration hits not only the vaguely remembered primal trauma and the undisposed-of anxiety representing it, but also a second trauma, consciously experienced and painful in character, though later obliterated by repression, namely weaning, the intensity and persistence of which falls far short of that of the first trauma, but owes a great part of its 'traumatic' effect to it. Only in the third place, then, does there appear the genital trauma of castration regularly phantasied in the history of the individual and, at most, experienced as a threat" (Rank, 1929, p. 21).
11 René Roussillon (2023): "It is a processual memory, a memory of sensations-forms-movements, a memory of interface encounters, a memory of contact, of a type of link, so it has neither subject nor object; it mixes the two since it is the meeting point between them. Processual memory traces are 'id' and 'not capable of becoming conscious in this form' (Freud, 1923)".

References

Auglagnier, P. (1975/2001). *The violence of interpretation: From pictogram to statement*, Trans. A. Sheridan. Routledge.

Bion, W.R. (1970). *Attention and interpretation*. Maresfield Library/Karnac.

Bion, W.R. (1975). *The grid and the caesura*. Karnac.

Bion, W.R. (1992). *Cogitations*. New extended edition. Karnac.

Freud, S. (1912). Recommendations to physicians practicing psycho-analysis. In *S.E.* (Vol. XII, pp. 109–120). Hogarth Press.

Freud, S. (1923). The ego and the id. In *S.E.* (Vol. XIX, pp. 3–66). Hogarth Press.

Freud, S. (1926). Inhibitions, symptoms and anxiety. In *S.E.* (Vol. XX, pp. 75–176). Hogarth Press.

Freud, S. (1933[1932]). The dissection of the psychical personality (New introductory lectures on psychoanalysis). In *S.E.* (Vol. XXII, p. 57–80). Hogarth Press.

Freud, S. (1941). Findings, ideas, problems. In *S.E.* (Vol. XXIII, pp. 299–300). Hogarth Press.

Fridman, W.H. (1991). *Le Cerveau Mobile, De l'immunité au système immunitaire*. Hermann.

Groddeck, G. (1923/1979). *The book of the It*, Trans. V.M.E. Collins. Vision Press Limited.

Pascal, B. (1670/1958). *Pascal's pensées*. E.P. Dutton. https://www.gutenberg.org/files/18269/18269-h/18269-h.htm?xid=PS_smithsonian

Rank, O. (1929). *The trauma of birth*. Harcourt, Brace & Company.

Roussillon, R. (2023). *Le besoin d'illusion: enjeux et conditions*. EPF Conference, Cannes, March 2023, pp. 4–5.

Shakespeare, W. (n.d.). Sonnet 65. In B. Mowat, P. Werstine, M. Poston, & R. Niles (Eds.), *The Folger Shakespeare library*. https://www.folger.edu/explore/shakespeares-works/shakespeares-sonnets/read/65/ (accessed June 26, 2024).

Acknowledgements

Our thanks to Howard B. Levine, Series Editor of the Routledge Wilfred R. Bion Studies Book Series, for his unflagging support and encouragement.

Chapter 1

The breath of life

Bion's concept of the proto-mental

Dolan Power

Introduction

My intention in this essay is to trace the history of Bion's use of his concept *proto-mental*, highlighting its initial introduction in his theorizing, through his development and use of the idea, and then to its apparent disappearance from his lexicon. Apparent in that its formal use as a specific term disappeared in his writings but the substance of its meaningfulness continued through to the end of his work. Despite this persistent meaningfulness, the concept of the proto-mental has been difficult for others to grasp and difficult for Bion to convey his intent in proposing the concept. This is best illustrated by the following excerpt from an audio recording taken from his seminar of July 4, 1978:

Q: [inaudible] … brought together two different concepts of yours—one, the beta element, and the other the protomental apparatus. I don't quite see how they wed with one another [inaudible] … only for evacuation, and now you seem to be talking about them as manifesting themselves in somatic phenomena, habits and things of that sort.

BION: I invented the term with the idea that it could be vacant, a space "to let", as it were, that could be borrowed for purposes of clarifying something or other. But there are things that do seem to me to suggest this combination of body and mind.(Bion, 2005, pp. 53–54)

I also review, discuss, and critique how subsequent writers have understood and discussed this concept and argued for its continued importance in psychoanalytic thinking and practice. I conclude the essay by arguing that Bion's concept of proto-mental articulates a level of human experience and functioning, and therefore clinical relevance, that highlights a sense of aliveness and vitality at a level of undifferentiation that distinguishes it from concepts such as beta, and container-contained phenomena. I also argue that this level of undifferentiated experience is related to difficulties in the countertransference when working analytically at the deepest levels of pathology.

DOI: 10.4324/9781003534365-1

Discussion of Bion's use of the term proto-mental

Over the course of Bion's professional life, he made two explicit references to the concept of the "proto-mental". His first reference is made in 1952 written in an article entitled "Group Dynamics: A Re-view". This article was an effort to delineate his ideas regarding basic assumptions operating in a group and their effect on the work task of the group. At a certain point he details the characteristics of the mental state involved in participating in group basic assumptions, contrasting it with the activity of group work tasks:

> Participation in basic assumption mental activity requires no training, experience or mental development. It is instantaneous, inevitable and instinctive. In contrast with W. [Work Group] it makes no demands on the individual for a capacity to co-operate but depends on the individual's possession of what I call valency—a term I borrow from the physicists to express a capacity for instantaneous involuntary combination of one individual with another for sharing and acting on a basic assumption.
>
> (Bion, 1952, p. 235)

In the above quote Bion describes a mental activity that requires no prior learning or experience. He characterizes this mental activity as a capacity that is "instantaneous, inevitable and instinctive" and primarily dependent on the "instantaneous involuntary combination of one individual with another". This leaves the reader with the impression of a spontaneous combustion happening between individuals that is immediate and preordained.

What is Bion talking about here? Shortly thereafter he introduces us to a specific term for what heretofore had been referred to in vaguer descriptive terms, as if he is presenting all parts of the elephant before naming the elephant. He names it now with the term the "proto-mental system" and defines it in the following way:

> To account for the fate of the inactive basic assumptions I have postulated the existence of a proto-mental system in which physical and mental activity is undifferentiated and which lies outside the field ordinarily considered profitable for psychological investigation.
>
> (Bion, 1952, p. 236)

Bion's second reference to "proto-mental" can be found in his book *Experience in Groups and Other Papers* (1961). In this publication he writes the following:

> What is the fate of the two basic assumptions that are not operative? I propose to link this question with the question left unanswered earlier

about the nature and origin of the combination in which emotions were held in their association with any basic assumption.

(p. 100)

I include the remainder of this quote, which, although lengthy, properly conveys Bion's intention and thought in writing about the proto-mental. It is this greater contextual meaning surrounding existing references to the proto-mental that often gets short shrift or entirely lost.

Bion continues:

I said then that there were no observations at present available to the psychiatrist to explain why emotions associated with a basic assumption were held in combination with each other with such tenacity and exclusiveness. In order to explain this linkage and at the same time to explain the fate of the inoperative basic assumptions, I propose to postulate the existence of "proto-mental" phenomena. I cannot represent my view adequately without proposing a concept that transcends experience. Clinically, I make a psychological approach, and therefore note phenomena only when they present themselves as psychological manifestations. Nevertheless, it is convenient to me to consider that the emotional state precedes the basic assumption and follows certain proto-mental phenomena of which it is an expression. Even this statement is objectionable because it establishes a more rigid order of cause and effect than I wish to subscribe to, for clinically it is useful to consider these events as links in a circular series; sometimes it is convenient to think that the basic assumption has been activated by consciously expressed thoughts, at others in strongly stirred emotions, the outcome of proto-mental activity. There is no harm in commencing the series where we choose if it throws light on what takes place.

(Bion, 1961, pp. 100–101)

Bion seems to be struggling to find a way to describe and to think about experience before it is apparent to the clinician as a psychological phenomenon. He is particularly focused on why certain feelings (basic assumptions) persistently adhere to one another. He is trying to answer the question of what happens to basic assumptions that are not being expressed. What is striking is how frustrated he feels in attempting to create a concept or term for this because it inevitably begins to assign sequential order to a concept that he considers more circular and in dynamic revolving movement. We continue to struggle with this problem with language and how to express psychoanalytic ideas even today. For instance, Goldberg (2019) in particular has offered an important corrective to an unintended way we can assign and value linear development in considering beta as more primitive until it has been rendered representation by alpha function.

From the inception his earliest use of the concept of the proto-mental Bion seemed to struggle with describing a dynamic but non-linear process. Unfortunately, when he dropped the term proto-mental and became more interested in beta elements and their transformation through alpha function, there was an implied closing down of his original wish to keep a circular quality active in the use of his terms and this emphasis on dynamic, non-linear, circularity seemed also to disappear. That is, the process of beta elements being transformed into alpha elements via the container-contained function is by definition a linear one. Losing sight of this circular active quality that Bion described in the quote above has been an unfortunate consequence of theorizing a linearity in the relationship between beta elements, alpha elements, and alpha function. This ordering implies a progressive and directional movement from bodily/primitive/sensorial experience to the theoretically higher and more valued (implicitly and explicitly) level of representation, words, and understanding (understanding as K in Bion's terms) supplied through alpha function. In this process equation, I would argue, Bion's original emphasis on active and non-linear circulation is lost.

Valency

When he first introduces his idea of the proto-mental, Bion employs the term *valency* to refer to a capacity for cooperative work in a group and which each member of a group possesses in varying degrees (Mawson, 2014, Vol. IV, p. 187). This capacity for cooperative work reflects an important quality of the proto-mental. Specifically, he describes valency as a:

> readiness to combine on levels that can hardly be called mental at all but are characterized by behavior in the human being that is more analogous to tropism in plants than to purposive behavior such as is implicit in a word like "assumption". In short, I wish to use it for events in the proto-mental (pm) system should need arise.
>
> (Mawson, 2014, Vol. XIV, p. 187).

Bion goes on to explain that he borrowed the term "valency" from physics to depict "a *capacity for instantaneous involuntary combination* [my emphasis] of one individual with another for sharing and acting on a basic assumption" (Mawson, 2014, Vol. IV, p. 217). Here Bion draws our attention to an aspect or layer of all human experience that is neither bodily nor mental but is instead a realm, always present in us, where experience is entirely undifferentiated. Is the threat of being confronted with this undifferentiated realm of experience one way to understand what he refers to later as the "emotional storm" that occurs whenever two people are in a room together (Bion, 1979, p. 321)? Bléandonu's (1994) seminal work on Bion's life and work emphasizes the importance Bion wished to place on an individual's capacity for combining and collaborating with others in a work group. Collaboration takes place on a more conscious level while valency or the capacity for combining happens out of awareness in the undifferentiated experience of the proto-mental. Bléandonu states: "an individual without valency would no longer be human" (Bléandonu, 1994, p. 72). This is a dramatic statement that brings to mind Winnicott's "there's no such thing as an infant, there's an infant and someone" (1960, footnote 4, p. 587) or Aulagnier's (1975, p. 25) poetic description of the importance of the mother's unconscious "irradiating" the infant and in this way igniting a sense of bodily self-experience of vitality and being alive.

Bion's emphasis on an *"involuntary combination"* shines a floodlight on a movement propensity in our psyche-soma/soma-psyche that is instinctual (body based), involuntary (nonconscious), and instantaneous (immediate); a propensity for "combustion" that ignites between individuals in a group. He likens this propensity to that of a chemical reaction or "tropism"; people turning toward/reacting to each other like plants turn instinctively toward light. Implied here is a life force that is not part of "mental life" nor is it part of our internalized world of objects, but rather is so elemental as to be best thought of as foundational to being human. While Bion was inspired by his mentor William Trotter he was also clear that he did not agree with Trotter's (1916) notion of herd instinct as a driving force operating between the individual and the group. Bion preferred to think of valency as a quality inherent in an individual's capacity for combining with others at an elemental undifferentiated level.

After 1961 Bion drops the term proto-mental from his theorizing and seems to shift his focus to beta elements and elaborating his thoughts on alpha function. He refers to "proto-thoughts" (1962) in describing the early stage or level of development in thinking and to "proto-resistance" as an early stage of analytic resistance. His use of the prefix "proto" in this way is in line with its frequent use in psychoanalytic literature to designate something earlier, less developed or more primitive and in need of transformation toward a state of higher structure, differentiation, symbolization, or representability.[1] The general inference being communicated to the reader is that the author is referring to something primitive and/or early in development. This is understandable since the origin of proto is Greek and means "first, source, parent preceding, earliest form, original, basic" (Etymonline, n.d.). The psychoanalytic tradition of attaching the prefix proto simply mirrors the general usage of attaching proto to imply first or early, i.e., protoplanet, protoplasm, or prototype to name a few.

Though understandable from this perspective, I would argue there was a subtle shift in Bion's use of the term of "proto" as he developed his theory further (i.e., as above in "proto-thoughts" [1962]), a shift that contributed to the loss of his original intentions when describing the proto-mental as a realm of experience where cause and effect, sequencing, linearity, and differentiation give way to the preeminent quality of dynamic, circular, and evolving movement. Left behind is Bion's original effort to describe this undifferentiated level of experience, a level that is ongoing and circulates between being backgrounded and then foregrounded and brought to greater activation.

The proto-mental system and beta elements

In hypothesizing the proto-mental realm Bion described experience that is not only mental and not only physical, but rather is *fundamentally other than* more articulated psychological/emotional/physical experience. His subsequent discovery of beta elements (and the alpha function through which these elements are transformed) raises a question: what is the relationship between these levels of experience?

Beta elements *evolve from* the protomental system but are *only part* of it. Bion stresses the circularity and ongoing qualities of the proto-mental system. This means a certain portion of it remains intact at an undifferentiated level even as part of it may become differentiated, and in doing so attain definition and status as beta elements. Furthermore, this movement in qualifying experience at the proto-mental level implies that beta elements may be more than bits of unmetabolized experience only fit for evacuation if they are not transformed by alpha function. Goldberg (2012, 2014, 2019, 2020) in particular has emphasized this latter point, arguing against an unintended bias in psychoanalytic thinking that somato-psychic experience is "less" or "more primitive" than alpha elements and their subsequent narrative representation (beta elements that have been transformed through alpha function). Instead, Goldberg (2019, p. 413) encourages us to give full credence to what he refers to as the "realm of sensation" and the "shared embodied domain" of experience as a vitalizing aspect inherently part of human experience. However, while Goldberg elevates the importance of beta elements in their own right (and importantly further defines the historically vague notion of "beta function"), he pays less attention to the ongoing contributions of proto-mental experience, equating it solely with early development:

> In this regard, reference to "proto-mental" states and phenomena can be misleading; insofar as the proto-mental tends to denote a developmentally earlier, primordial or preliminary level of mental functioning, this should not be confused with the sensory pattern language which, as I have suggested, exists in its own right as a full-fledged type of psychical functioning, one that presents itself in the form of embodied being-in-the-world, rather than an immature form of mental life requiring transformation into symbolic thought for its effect.
>
> (Goldberg, 2019, p. 413)

I would argue a different view however, one I believe is more consistent with the overall sensibility and trajectory of Bion's thought (Vermote, 2019, pp. 62–63) and maintain that beta elements derive from a *part* of the proto-mental system but should not be equated with its entirety (see also Cartwright, 2010, p. 109, and Meltzer, 1986, p. 12).

Viewed this way proto-mental phenomena are always somewhere in the present providing a crucial foundational *matrix* that enables the eventual agglomeration of what we can call, following Goldberg (2019), *embodied, sensorial beta experience*. Such a perspective preserves Bion's proto-mental as a dimension of experience coincident with beta and alpha function and operating in the circulating motion Bion originally proposed. Further, it preserves Bion's original intent to "let" space for the ongoing presence of the proto-mental even when it is momentarily backgrounded and counters its dismissal as an immature or primitive stage of somatopsychic life. In this way, we avoid the conceptual flaw inherent in imagining development as an arrangement of linear stages or levels of organization (especially stages of representability) and retain instead a view of human experience as more nuanced, dynamic, and complex, a view more consistent with contemporary psychoanalytic thinking. All three modes of experience (the proto-mental, beta and alpha function) exist although at any given moment one or more of them may be backgrounded as future potentials or silent capacities. This line of thought naturally suggests that the instantaneous, undifferentiated proto-mental experience, whereby definition inside and outside are not differentiated, is different from beta experience which tends to have a clearer location in the body and the perceptual apparatus.

Post Bionian views of the concept of the proto-mental

Several psychoanalytic writers have held on to Bion's original thoughts concerning the proto-mental system while productively elaborating his ideas and applying them to psychoanalytic technique. Central among these authors are Donald Meltzer (1986), Claudio Neri (1993), Duncan Cartwright (2010, 2016), and Rudi Vermote (2011, 2013, 2019).

Donald Meltzer emphasized the importance of Bion's proto-mental system, devoting an entire chapter to elaborating its clinical manifestations in his 1986 book *Studies in Extended Metapsychology*. He considered the interplay between the mental and the proto-mental fundamental to development and connects their back and forth to a "competition for the child's soul" (Meltzer, 1986, p. 12). Meltzer interprets Bion's view of development not in the usual way of including the achievement of a series of steps or stages of development but involving the viewpoint that development is happiness. Meltzer disagrees with the psychoanalytic literature's emphasis on growth being primarily and inevitably tied to a balance of pain and pleasure. Meltzer emphasizes that for Bion an individual's development and happiness "requires learning from experience" and the "traversing of catastrophic change" (1986, p. 12). Here he is reframing more traditional psychoanalytic views of psychosexual development in preference for how the proto-mental level and its ongoing involvement with bodily development influences the structuring of the self. This line of thought views the embryonic and pre-natal periods as having important contributions to the post-natal self and experience.

Williams, in her introduction to *Studies in Extended Metapsychology*, goes so far as to state that distinguishing between the proto-mental and truly mental or symbolic levels of the mind is the central organizing principle to Meltzer's view of psychoanalytic work. She goes on to explain his view that the "caesura between them [the proto-mental and the symbolic capacities—author's note] relates back to prenatal life and soma-psychotic states which become fossilized if ignored by postnatal parts of the personality" (Meltzer, 1986, p. xii). The inference here is that a nascent self is beginning to form in the womb and that difficulty can be brought into post-natal life via the proto-mental level which contains a "seed of the pre-natal conjecture" (Mawson, 2011, p. 126) ripe with potentialities. Mawson ponders, "how can we build in psychoanalysis receptive screens for containing these emotional pre-natal forces, in a similar way as artists do when they build forms that catch the 'light', generating more light than heat?" (Mawson, 2011, p. 127). For the personality, and as Mawson suggests also for the analyst and her theories, the basic tension here is between the undifferentiated proto-mental level and the progressive ability to differentiate via evolving beta elements and alpha function. Following Meltzer's line of thinking we might conclude, clinically, it is this tension that underlies the analyst's struggle to contain counter-transference experience when working with more disturbed patients who operate on the more undifferentiated level of the proto-mental. It is a struggle experienced at an individual level and also at a professional level within psychoanalysis: how do we remain open and receptive to the proto-mental registration of experience without obliterating it through an overly active effort to "capture it" through interpretation or through overly "organizing experience" with a linear understanding of psychological development and life? Do our efforts clinically to find and offer "representations" of our encounters with this dimension of intersubjective engagement sometimes reflect a defensive need to give form to that which is formless?

In 1993 Claudio Neri wrote about the proto-mental system and connected this concept to an ongoing part of individual experience and subjectivation. In an article linking the proto-mental level to the transgenerational transmission of trauma he described the process of transmission as one that is closer to "gases" that pass through individuals wafting from one generation to the next. Additionally, he uses words like "diffuse", "impalpable", "formless", and "ubiquitous", to further describe the qualities of what is being handed down from one generation to another (Neri, 1993, pp. 47–48). Neri offers us an image of the intergenerational transmission of trauma founded on a porosity of experience, where the mental and physical are undifferentiated, hence implicating involvement at the proto-mental level. Neri's is a very different way to conceptualize the transmission process and does not include imagining one person identifying with well-defined or specific characteristics of others. It is not built on a model of identification. But if not transmission via our usual models of identificatory processes, how do we understand the kind of transmission Neri's image is trying to capture? The natural world may offer us some help here. For example, consider the phenomenon of "murmuration" commonly seen in the behavior of European starlings in flight where waves of undulating flight patterns unfold seemingly as magic, the birds appearing to be one giant pulsating organism rather than a group of individual birds, and where it is not possible to discern who is initiating shifts in the unfolding patterns. Likewise, schools of reef fish can suggest this same type of functioning, visually suggestive of the tropistic nature of the proto-mental— exemplifying a high degree of valency—the capacity to combine with another so powerfully on display. Neri is suggesting a similar process may be at play in the transgenerational transmission of trauma and that this operates non-consciously at the proto-mental level. This doesn't preclude the possibility of unconscious contributions to the transmission process but only adds a different kind of transmission process originating from this undifferentiated level of experience.

Neri asks if the analyst's effort to stay alive during difficult periods of analytic work is part of holding onto one's subjectivity in the presence of a fusional pull of the proto-mental level. At an undifferentiated level where the psychological and the physical are felt to be one and the same, does staying alive and separate become threatened by a pull toward undifferentiated experience?

In his book *Containing States of Mind*, Duncan Cartwright (2010) brings both a clarity of thought and an accessible writing style to the articulation of Bion's concept of the proto-mental. Cartwright defines basic assumptions as "prototypical organizing principles that are inseparable from each other" (Cartwright, 2010, p. 118) and that are like "the capillary blood system that responds to external conditions by dilating or lying dormant" (Cartwright, 2010, p. 109). With this additional image, he offers us his articulation of Bion's tropism, a valency characteristic of the proto-mental system. Cartwright emphasizes the point that Bion is talking about an area of experience that is inherently human and thus preexisting, and which contains emergent properties that are further differentiated via interaction with the external world. For Bion this proto-mental area implies an experience "where the individual is as much 'in the group' as the group is 'in the individual'" (Cartwright, 2010, p. 109). Cartwright connects the proto-mental to Bourdieu's (1997) sociological term "habitus" which refers to the idea that what we mean by "culture" is the everyday aspects of individual and group life that are embedded in the body. Bourdieu refers to this more specifically as "a generative principle of regulated improvisations" (Bourdieu, 1997, p. 78) that have an "intentionless invention" (Bourdieu, 1997, p. 79). In this it is easy to hear a resonance with Meltzer's (1986, p. 12) description of the proto-mental qualities of "habitual, automatic, unintentional". Cartwright goes on to suggest that counter to Winnicott's (1971/2005, p. 176) idea of "being before doing", proto-mental functioning is dependent upon "doing before being": "actions-movement systems do not occur in isolation of an interpersonal context so it appears more accurate to a 'doing together' that is generated at a non-conscious level" (Cartwright, 2010, p. 117).

Rudi Vermote has elaborated on the theoretical and clinical relevance of the proto-mental system (2013, 2019) and in doing so emphasizes that it is omnipresent in analytic process. The challenge is to access this level since at the level of our represented experience (images and words) we are not necessarily in contact with the proto-mental and functioning at this more symbolically organized level of experience may unintentionally obstruct contact with this more undifferentiated level of experience. Vermote states that while Bion dropped the term proto-mental after 1961 he returned to its importance in his later writings. During this period, often referred to by Vermote (2011, p. 1098) as "late Bion", he was interested in how to generate a sense of aliveness, recognizing that adherence to abstract theories and intellectualized understanding can deaden vitality and the growth-promoting aspects of any psychoanalytic process. Vermote points to the importance Bion placed on transformations in hallucinosis (Bion, 1965, p. 134) and links this to a rebirth of Bion's interest in the undifferentiated level of proto-mental experience. In this way he connects Bion's later writings and references to an undifferentiated level of experience to Bion's concept of at-one-ment. Vermote (2013, p. 16) places special emphasis on the ongoing paradox he finds in Bion's thinking: some undifferentiated experience requires transformation by the analyst's alpha function as a vital part of responding to some forms of pathology—while at the same time considering the proto-mental level as a constant level of undifferentiated experience providing a fundamental source of creativity and sense of being alive.

Discussion of Bion's proto-mental and the implications for psychoanalytic theory

I will now summarize and discuss five aspects of the concept of proto-mental experience that highlight both its confusing presence in psychoanalytic literature as well as its potential contributions to our contemporary interest in nonconscious, unrepresented, and inter-corporeal experience.

First, there has been an unintentional tendency to put a form (i.e., give qualities) to the proto-mental by referring to it as the body, or raw internal or somatic sensations. Bion's concern in creating this concept is that it would be misunderstood in just this way. He feared that giving it this kind of conceptual form would foreclose understanding of the foundational and undifferentiated quality of what he referred to as the proto-mental. His wish was to characterize it as a "circulating" experience where basic assumptions (feelings) rotated forward in consciousness while other basic assumptions receded into the proto-mental matrix but did not disappear. Bion tried to elucidate the proto-mental by likening it to the tropism of plants that turn toward light. He wanted a concept that suggested a foundational state of being but that could also be kept open and unsaturated of meaning. Bion's emphasis was always on movement, circularity, porosity, and permeability, rather than on anchoring the concept in a particular bodily or sensory experience.

Secondly, there is a confusing tendency to equate the proto-mental with "primitive experience", an equation which may stem from its being undifferentiated and non-symbolized. As I have outlined above, Bion's original intent was to describe a foundational state of being (foundational while not primitive, and where inside and outside is not differentiated), an intention that remained unaltered throughout the corpus of his work.

Thirdly, we should continue to distinguish Bion's concept of the proto-mental from other useful concepts but which describe intersubjective processes. By contrast for example, Ogden's (2004) concept of the intersubjective third requires the unconscious contributions from two separate subjectivities.

But if not intersubjective, how can we usefully imagine its mode of expression? I have suggested above several examples from the natural world (starlings, reef fish) that may offer us some assistance in so doing. De Toffolli (2011) offers us yet another example of what the philosopher Daniel Dennet described as an "intuition pump" (Dennett, 1997).[2] In discussing modes of bodily experience, she describes how food and feeding models have been used in conceptualizing the psychoanalytic relationship. She notes however that respiratory models as such have remained largely on the periphery and are seldom, if ever, invoked in these types of discussions. I think her description of breathing provides us with a beautiful metaphor for Bion's proto-mental:

> breathing is not a voluntary act; the biochemical transformations that characterize it are not under our control. When air enters the lungs of one individual, it pervades his or her body, leaves it, and potentially circulates in the body of another individual, outside of our consciousness or our perception. Moreover, air spreads throughout the whole body, the breath coinciding with the body's life. But—in contrast to the situation with food—breath goes beyond the body and is not in itself containable; it moves freely I to you….
>
> (de Toffolli, 2011, p. 602)[3]

Here breathing is commensurate with a foundational flow of experience or breath of life that is a constant. It does not require transformation into a "higher" form of psychological functioning but provides the life supporting undercurrent for all forms of more differentiated psychological and physical experience. It is not under conscious control and is not given by one individual to another as is suggested by a metaphor of mother/analyst feeding the infant/patient. It is not a thing to be given or taken in by separate individuals but better thought of as a flow of being-as-breathing.

Fourthly, there is a tendency to equate the proto-mental with beta elements, or perhaps even retire the term proto-mental entirely in preference for beta elements. Rather than opt for either of these choices I suggest instead that there is benefit in differentiating non-symbolic processes into two separate categories: the proto-mental and beta elements. This line of thinking is consistent with Cartwright (2010), who infers from Bion (1961, p. 153) that beta elements arise from the proto-mental but should not be equated with the proto-mental:

> He [Bion] seems to be suggesting here that this is akin to joining a field of experience that is already there. The above appears to suggest that proto-mental systems of which beta elements are a part may have self-organizing capacities.
>
> (Cartwright, 2010, pp. 107–109)

Often psychoanalytic theories have tended to break down around a mind body dualism, leaving us with an opposition of bodily or somatic experience vs symbolic thought and where health becomes synonymous with the capacity to represent somatic experience (transform it into symbolic form). Cartwright (2010) and other contemporary authors (de Toffoli, 2011; Goldberg, 2019; Pelz, 2014; Vermote, 2011, 2016) are forging a new path regarding unrepresented experience in general, arguing for the necessary presence of sub-symbolic experience in healthy living. In common, these writers recognize and legitimize the presence of nonconscious and unrepresented experience in both patient and analyst. With this in mind I suggest we avoid simply abandoning the concept of the proto-mental and maintain instead the view stated above, namely that beta elements arise out of the proto-mental *but without assigning value or linearity to this process.* From this perspective proto-mental life is something akin to a background state of being that remains undifferentiated, elemental to being alive and closer to what Matte-Blanco described as infinite experience (Raynor & Tuckett, 1988, p. 40). The term "infinite" here carrying an inherent meaning of unlimited potential or emergent capacity. Viewed as originating from the ongoing circulation of proto-mental experience, beta elements (accretions of stimuli that are agglomerated) then become more specific expressions of experience or behavior which add color and texture to life. This model avoids the problem of lumping together what should be viewed as two different types of unrepresented experience.

Why maintain this distinction? Recall for instance the metaphors de Toffoli (2011) offers us in which she distinguishes the involuntary nature of respiratory exchanges from the more intentional experience of nutritional exchanges involving food. Similarly, proto-mental experience, tropistic and instantaneous, is commensurate with breathing in that it is nonconscious and is synonymous with life, circulates freely from outside to inside and back out to another's inside. This circulation happening between inside and outside and within the individual is not voluntary, and neither is any exchange between individuals. Here the mechanism of exchange and what is being exchanged are not sensorially perceptible and the exchange is a freely ongoing one in a two-way direction. By comparison, beta elements are related to sensorial experience and in this way are part of the perceptual system of hearing, seeing, tasting, touch, and smell. And finally, beta elements are differentiated (hence the word "elements") while Bion likened the proto-mental to the body's capillary action, and in that sense to an undifferentiated flow.

Although Bion sometimes appeared to have moved away from his early thoughts regarding the proto-mental, he goes out of his way in a 1971 Los Angeles lecture on the grid to make a plea for open mindedness amongst psychoanalysts regarding something basic and mysterious operating within each analysand:

> Sometimes it becomes clear to the psychoanalyst that the boundaries do not correspond to the person's anatomical structure. Melanie Klein, as I understand her to say, did not think there was any mystery about apparently concerted movements in a group of analysands beyond what could be explained by transference relationship with the same analyst. I think we should keep an open mind. I do not feel any need to postulate "extra-sensory" perception, a herd instinct as Wilfred Trotter did, or a group unconscious as Jung did. I think, however, that there may well be some analogue in the personality to the capillary blood system which in ordinary conditions is dormant but in extraordinary conditions may dilate as in surgical shock.
>
> (Mawson, 2014, Vol. X, p. 24)

Lastly, proto-mental experience is often associated in our literature with pre-natal experience (Vermote, 2019, p. 184) and also with late Bion's (Vermote, 2011, 2019) introduction of the concept of O. Vermote (2013, p. 16) summarizes the impact of Bion's evolving thoughts on the proto-mental as including a central paradox. Is undifferentiated, formless experience inherently part of severe pathology and, therefore, in need of transformation? Or, is undifferentiated, formless experience a prerequisite for creativity and a life-giving necessity for health? Vermote encourages us to keep both views in mind and to tolerate the inherent contradiction implied by these questions.

Bion's concept of the proto-mental affords the psychoanalyst an imaginative tool for conceiving a quality of human experience where even our language for describing forms of relatedness is challenged since our language, including the word "relatedness" itself, immediately constrains and delimits the very qualities of experience we are trying to capture. In the presence of the kind of undifferentiated experiences we are so often confronted with clinically, our language of self and object can become awkward in the extreme. I would argue that conceptualizing certain aspects of experience as nested in the proto-mental matrix offers both further support and language to investigations into pre-natal experience, early post-natal life, states of being in which psychic vitality itself is threatened, our current interest in inter-corporeality, difficult countertransference situations, and many other areas of contemporary psychoanalytic interest.

Final thoughts

Cartwright (2016, p. 207) states that "there are no caesuras in the proto-mental system". Rather, there is an undifferentiated experience of a "sense of flow" or "moving along" where sound is like sonar and rhythmic pressures of being encourage the flow of potential and the possibility of something emerging out of nothing. Giving credence to this aspect of pre-natal experience recognizes the important foundational experience of this undifferentiated beginning to life out of which develops a background state of being that remains a constant throughout life. This background state of being allows the various potentials to eventually agglomerate as beta elements while a portion of the proto-mental continues the necessary circulation of breath that sustains a sense of involuntary aliveness. While these ideas regarding the proto-mental can take on a somewhat poetic lilt, I suggest that whatever lack of specificity we might find in them reflects the very formlessness of the experience itself, leaving us only our intuition pumps as a tool for capturing what is by its very nature evanescent.

In elaborating his ideas regarding pre-natal life in Caesura (Mawson, 2014, Vol. X, p. 35) Bion drew on Freud (1926) for support: "there is much more continuity between intra-uterine life and earliest infancy than the impressive caesura of the act of birth allows us to believe" (Freud, 1926, p. 138). Pistiner de Cortinas (2011, p. 129f) notes that Bion believed there was a prevailing operant bias that favored "consciously known functioning, we are also blind to our proto-mental or pre-natal manifestations". Bion felt that Freud was in error in not pursuing a deeper understanding of the continuity between pre-natal and post-natal life (Bion, 2000, p. 271). Often these proto-mental and pre-natal manifestations are experienced by the analyst as distracting obstacles to our preferred methods for achieving psychoanalytic understanding. Yet, it is obvious that Bion's concept of the pre-natals (*Memoir of the Future*, 1977/1991) references not only a gestational period prior to birth but also to ongoing potentials inherently available in the proto-mental matrix throughout life, awaiting possible psychological birth.

During a discussion held at the VA Hospital in Brentwood, Los Angeles in 1976, Bion lamented to the audience of young clinicians: "I wonder when the psychiatrists and psycho-analysts will catch up with the foetus. When will *they* be able to hear and see these things [that the foetus sees and hears]?" (Bion, 2000, p. 274). With this question Bion tasks psychoanalysts to be open to an undifferentiated proto-mental experience that is easily lost or closed off with words and mental images. Later in the same year he published an essay entitled "Evidence" in the Bulletin of the British Psychoanalytical Society in which he elaborated on the importance of what the analyst hears and sees of the unknown:

> It may be the case that we are here dealing with things that are so slight as to be virtually imperceptible, but so real that they could destroy us almost without our being aware of it. *That* is the kind of area into which we have to penetrate.
>
> (Mawson, 2014, Vol. IV, p. 135)

Toward the end of his career Bion asked, "will psychoanalysis study the living mind?" (Bion, 1979, p. 330) This was a question that evolved for him over time and can be linked to his interest in the proto-mental matrix (1961, *Experience in Groups*), to his interest in hallucinosis (1967, *Second Thoughts*), and finally to his interest in the pre-natal (*Memoir of the Future*, 1977/1991). The underlying thread connecting these areas of thought can be found in his pursuit of an undifferentiated area of experience and linking it to the life-giving world inherent in an elemental state of being of the proto-mental (Grotstein, 2007; Vermote, 2011, 2013).

Notes

1 See for instance such terms as protoemotions (Civitarese, 2008; Ferro, 1996, 2002, 2003, 2005, 2006a, 2006b, 2009); proto-objectal (Sasso, 2021), proto-psychic (Civitarese, 2020), proto-container (Birksted-Breen, 2019; Molinari, 2020), proto-elements (Botella & Botella, 2005; Ithier, 2020), protoexperience (Blass, 2016, 2018; Greenberg, 2015; Raphael-Leff, 2013).
2 An intuition pump is "*not* supposed to clothe strict arguments that prove conclusions from premises. Rather, their point is to entrain a family of imaginative reflections in the reader that ultimately yields not a formal conclusion but a 'dictate' of intuition" (p. 12).
3 Note that the phrase "it moves freely I to you" denotes intentionless motion and does not imply evacuation in the psychoanalytic sense or projection, nor is it intended to suggest a container-contained relationship.

References

Aulagnier, P. (1975/2001). *The violence of interpretation: From pictogram to statement*, Trans. A. Sheridan. Routledge.

Bion, W.R. (1952). Group dynamics: A re-view. *International Journal of Psychoanalysis*, 33, 235–247.

Bion, W.R. (1961). *Experiences in groups and other papers*. Karnac.

Bion, W.R. (1962). *Learning from experience*. Karnac.

Bion, W.R. (1965). *Transformations: Change from learning to growth*. Karnac.

Bion, W.R. (1967/2018). *Second thoughts: Selected papers on psychoanalysis*. Routledge.

Bion, W.R. (1977/1991). *A memoir of the future*. Karnac.

Bion, W.R. (1979). Making the best of a bad job. In *Clinical seminars and other works*. Karnac.

Bion, W.R. (2000). *Clinical seminars and other works*. Ed. F. Bion. Karnac.

Bion, W.R. (2005). *The Tavistock seminars: Wilfred R. Bion*. Ed. F. Bion. Karnac.

Birksted-Breen, D. (2019). Pathways of the unconscious: When the body is the receiver/instrument. *International Journal of Psychoanalysis*, 100, 1117–1133.

Blass, R.B. (2016). The quest for truth as the foundation of psychoanalytic practice: A traditional Freudian-Kleinian perspective. *Psychoanalytic Quarterly*, 85, 305–337.

Blass, R.B. (2018). Introduction to "A Special Section on Lectures on Technique by Melanie Klein". *International Journal of Psychoanalysis*, 99, 947–951.

Bléandonu, G. (1994). *Wilfred Bion: His life and works 1897–1979*. Other Press.

Botella, C., & Botella, S. (2005). *The work of psychic figurability without representation*, Trans. A. Weller & M. Zerbib. The New Library of Psychoanalysis. Routledge.

Bourdieu, P. (1997). *The logic of practice*. Polity Press.

Cartwright, D. (2010). *Containing states of mind*. Routledge.

Cartwright, D. (2016). Containing systems in the analytic field. In H.B. Levine & G. Civitarese (Eds.), *The W.R. Bion tradition* (pp. 201–222). Karnac.

Civitarese, G. (2008). Immersion versus interactivity and the analytic field. *International Journal of Psychoanalysis*, 89, 279–298.

Civitarese, G. (2020). Regression in the analytic field. *Revue Roumaine de Psychanalyse*, 13, 17–41.

Dennett, D. (1997). *Elbow room: The varieties of free will worth wanting*. The MIT Press.

de Toffoli, C. (2011). The living body in the psychoanalytic experience. *Psychoanalytic Quarterly*, 80, 595–618.

Etymonline. (n.d.). Proto. https://www.etymonline.com/word/proto-#etymonline_v_2734

Ferro, A. (1996). Carla's panic attacks: Insight and transformation. *International Journal of Psychoanalysis*, 77, 997–1011.

Ferro, A. (2002). Superego transformations through the analyst's capacity for reverie. *Psychoanalytic Quarterly*, 77, 477–501.

Ferro, A. (2003). Marcella: The transition from explosive sensoriality to the ability to think. *Psychoanalytic Quarterly*, 72, 183–200.

Ferro, A. (2005). Which reality in the psychoanalytic session? *Psychoanalytic Quarterly*, 74, 421–442.

Ferro, A. (2006a). Clinical implications of Bion's thought. *International Journal of Psychoanalysis*, 87, 989–1003.

Ferro, A. (2006b). Trauma, reverie, and the field. *Psychoanalytic Quarterly*, 75, 1045–1056.

Ferro, A. (2009). Transformations in dreaming and characters in the psychoanalytic field. *International Journal of Psychoanalysis*, 90, 209–230.

Freud, S. (1926). Inhibitions, symptoms and anxiety. In *Standard edition* (vol. 20). Hogarth Press [originally published 1959].

Goldberg, P. (2012). Active perception and the search for sensory symbiosis. *JAPA*, 60, 791–812.

Goldberg, P. (2014). Containing states of mind: Exploring Bion's container model in psychoanalytic psychotherapy by Duncan Cartwright, Routledge, 2009. *Fort Da*, 20, 115–127.

Goldberg, P. (2019). Where are we when we are at one? Discussion of Bion's O and his pseudo-mystical path. *Psychoanalytic Dialogues*, 29, 404–417.

Goldberg, P. (2020). Body-mind dissociation, altered states, altered worlds. *Journal of the American Psychoanalytic Association*, 68, 769–806.

Greenberg, J. (2015). Therapeutic action and the analyst's responsibility. *Journal of the American Psychoanalytic Association*, 63, 15–32.

Grotstein, J.S. (2007). *A beam of intense darkness*. Routledge.

Ithier, B. (2020). Boundaries and depths of the oneiric. *International Journal of Psychoanalysis*, 101, 879–899.

Mawson, C. (Ed.) (2011). *Bion today*. Routledge.

Mawson, C. (Ed.) (2014). *The complete works of Wilfred R. Bion*. Karnac.

Meltzer, D. (1986). *Studies in extended metapsychology*. Karnac.

Molinari, E. (2020). Intimacy and autism: An apparent paradox. *Psychoanalytic Quarterly*, 89, 483–502.

Neri, C. (1993). Field theory and trans-generational phantasies. *Rivista di Psicoanalisi*, 39(1), 43–62.

Ogden, T.H. (2004). The analytic third: Implications for psychoanalytic theory and technique. *Psychoanalytic Quarterly*, 73, 167–195.

Peltz, R. (2014). Our bodies, ourselves, and the world: An introduction to Merlau-Ponty's philosophy of inter-corporeality. *Fort Da*, 20A(1), 30–32.

Pistiner de Cortinas, L. (2011). Science and fiction in the psychoanalytical field. In C. Mawson (Ed.), *Bion today*. Routledge.

Raphael-Leff, J. (2013). Psychic "geodes"—the presence of Absence: 18th Enid Balint Memorial Lecture, 2013. *Couple and Family Psychoanalysis*, 11, 299–315.

Raynor, E., & Tuckett, D. (1988). An introduction to Matte-Blanco's reformulation of the Freudian unconscious and his conceptualization of the internal world. In *Thinking, feeling, and being: Clinical reflections on the fundamental antimony of human beings and world*. The New Library of Psychoanalysis (Vol. 5). Routledge.

Sasso, G. (2021). The psychoanalysis-neurosciences interface: A proposal for a hypothetical unification of psychoanalytic models. *International Journal of Psychoanalysis*, 102, 68–90.

Trotter, W. (1916). *Instincts of the Herd in Peace and War*. Unwin.

Vermote, R. (2011). On the value of 'late Bion' to analytic theory and practice. *International Journal of Psychoanalysis*, 92, 1089–1098.

Vermote, R. (2013). The undifferentiated zone of psychic functioning: An integrative approach and clinical implication. *European Psychoanalytic Federation Bulletin*, 67, 16–27.

Vermote, R. (2016). On Bion's text "Emotional Turbulence": A focus on experience and the unknown. In H.B. Levine & G. Civitarese (Eds.), *The W.R. Bion tradition* (pp. 345–351). Karnac.

Vermote, R. (2019). *Reading Bion*. The New Library of Psychoanalysis. Routledge.

Winnicott, D.W. (1971/2005). *Playing and reality*. Routledge.

Winnicott, D.W. (1960). The theory of the parent infant relationship. *International Journal of Psychoanalysis*, 41, 585–595.

Chapter 2

Circling the nameless

An attempt at an impossible approach

Bernd Nissen

The nameless has no name and yet it is on everyone's lips these days. There are many attempts to give these conditions a name: e.g. nameless dread (Bion, e.g. 1962a, p. 96; 1962b, p. 309), breakdown (Winnicott, 1974), non-existent (Bion, 1970; Winnicott, 1974), or the more clinical term 'black hole' (Tustin, 1988), or 'deathscapes' (Benedetti, 1983). But it is not possible to find an empirically saturated name, it would be a contradictio in adiecto. This work attempts to approach the nameless theoretically—but cannot do without metapsychological speculation—and clinically. It is an impossible undertaking, but worth a try.

Starter: Short clinical example

Let's start circling around with a small clinical example:[1] a patient, Mrs. A., reported in the initial interview that she had developed a "perversion". Her perversion consisted of finding feces a source of sexual arousal. She ate her stool and smeared her whole body with feces and urine. On two occasions, she incurred a severe infection from these practices, and on one occasion it was life-threatening. The perversion was practiced alone but also with other frequently changing objects who did not, as she explained to me, "matter as persons or individuals". In these states of arousal, she frequently had anal intercourse without protection. At the same time, she suffered from inflammatory bowel disorders, causing diarrhea and frequent visits to the toilet. What is important now is this: these messages did not trigger anything in me, did not touch me. Even a weak background noise of defensive forces in me, as an indication of my involvement, was not discernible. If, for example, a colleague had recounted this material in a supervision session, aversive reactions (disgust, repulsion, etc.) would have been immediate. Although data are clearly named, they do not exist psychically, they have no name, no psychic meaning, hardly any sensual existence. They are nameless.

DOI: 10.4324/9781003534365-2

Basic theoretical considerations[2]

Bion writes about the nameless:

> Normal development follows if the relationship between infant and breast permits the infant to project a feeling, say, that it is dying, into the mother and to reintroject it after its sojourn in the breast has made it tolerable to the infant psyche. If the projection is not accepted by the mother the infant feels that its feeling that it is dying is stripped of such meaning as it has. It therefore reintrojects, not a fear of dying made tolerable, but a nameless dread.
>
> (1962b, p. 309; see 1962a, p. 96)

Nameless dread results from a failed projection and introjection dynamic in which meaning is "withdrawn". But what is happening in the relationship and what is being withdrawn?

The psychic and its qualities

In his work on thinking, Bion operates with two concepts of consciousness: a consciousness that depends on alpha-function and a restricted term of "limited consciousness": "the limited consciousness defined by Freud, that I am using to define a rudimentary infant consciousness, is not associated with an unconscious. All impressions of the self are of equal value; all are conscious" (Bion, 1962b, p. 309). This "consciousness produces 'sense-data' of the self, but that there is no alpha-function to convert them into alpha-elements and therefore permit of a capacity for being conscious or unconscious of the self" (1962b, p. 308f).[3]

It is a pure perception consciousness that notices internal and external impressions and sensations without perceiving the *psychic* qualities. Here the α-function comes into play: "alpha-function operates on the sense impressions, whatever they are, and the emotions, whatever they are, of which the patient is *aware*" (1962a, p. 6; italics BN),[4] i.e. inner and outer impressions which are captured by the perception consciousness are qualified by the α-function and become α-elements. "These elements are suited to storage and the requirements of dream thoughts" (1962a, p. 6) of waking life or sleep. If the sense impressions and sensations are not "digested" by the α-function, they become β-elements (see 1962a).[5]

Initially, the mother in her reverie takes on this function for the infant, who communicates its states to the mother via projective identification.

> As a *realistic* activity it shows itself as behaviour reasonably calculated to arouse in the mother feelings of which the infant wishes to be rid. If the infant feels it is dying it can arouse fears that it is dying in the mother. A

well-balanced mother can accept these and respond therapeutically: that is to say in a manner that makes the infant feel it is receiving its frightened personality back again, but in a form that it can tolerate—the fears are manageable by the infant personality.

(1962b, p. 308)

This means that the fear of death is qualified and made bearable. But Bion is not only operating with a model in which unbearable conditions become bearable, but also with a relational-serial one; in "Elements of Psychoanalysis", he writes:

the infant, filled with painful lumps of faeces, guilt, fears of impending death, chunks of greed, meanness and urine, evacuates these bad objects into the breast that is not there. As it does so the good object turns the no-breast (mouth) into a breast, the faeces and urine into milk, the fears of impending death and anxiety into vitality and confidence, the greed and meanness into feelings of love and generosity and the infant sucks its bad property, now translated into goodness, back again.

(1963, p. 31)

That means two things: on the one hand, nameless fear of dying, for example, is transformed into bearable fear, on the other hand, dreadful hunger can be replaced by blissful satisfaction. The states on which the α-function has an effect exist eo ipso and do not depend on a relational transformation—even if they are related in the psychic structure. The resulting elements are thus differentiated and related in themselves. With the re-introjection, not only α-elements are internalized but also functional ability.

We are here on the level of sense impressions and sensations, which are qualified by the α-function. But do they already have psychic quality?

I think the answer is quite clear: probably not. Bion writes that the psychoanalyst is dependent

on experience that is not sensuous.... The realizations with which a psycho-analyst deals cannot be seen or touched; anxiety has no shape or colour, smell or sound. For convenience, I propose to use the term 'intuit' as a parallel in the psychoanalyst's domain to the physician's use of 'see', 'touch', 'smell', and 'hear'.

(1970, p. 7)

The psychic is not sensuous in essence, can only be intuited. Only through the secondary qualities, as we have just derived them, can they be known (K):

Thoughts have as their background realizations that are sensible: anxiety, fear, sex can be thought about only when O has evolved to a point where it is apprehensible in sense and has become amenable to transformations in K. Anxiety is 'known' by its secondary qualities. Yet no one has any doubt about anxiety or about 'feeling' the reality, though what is felt is sensations associated with anxiety and not anxiety itself.

(1970, p. 35)

I.e., the psychic can be known through the "secondary" qualities, in other words through qualified sensory impressions (K), but in its core dimension (the "psychic itself") it is not sensual, can only be intuited, and shows itself at the moment of its realization. But without relationship this process cannot be thought, indeed the child existentially needs the mother. How is the relation between realization and relationship to be understood?

Freud (e.g. 1915) develops his psychology from the components of affect and (re)presentation. I think Bion follows him. He formulates the nature of a psychoanalytical object as follows:

Suppose ψ represents a constant, (ξ) an unsaturated element that determines the value of the constant once it has been identified. We may use the unknown constant ψ to represent an inborn pre-conception. Employing a model to give temporary meaning to the term "inborn pre-conception" I shall suppose that an infant has an inborn pre-conception that a breast that satisfies its own incomplete nature exists. The realization of the breast provides an emotional experience. This experience corresponds to Kant's secondary and primary qualities of a phenomenon. The secondary qualities determine the value of the unsaturated element (ξ) and therefore the value of ψ (ξ). This sign now represents a conception.

(Bion, 1962a, p. 69)[6]

The "hardly definable knowledge" (Freud) that something exists (e.g. what we call "breast") is the unknown that we also have to intuit. This intuition is on both sides of O, before the moment of presence and after the moment of presence in which the realization occurs (see below).

The pre-conception has two very important features: 1. It has an *objectal structure*. The infant has a preparatory of the breast and is able to arouse states of expectation in the mother. And the mother, with her developed psychic apparatus, has a pre-conception too. She is expecting her child and can react appropriately. The expectation of the pre-conception "breast" is the *expectation of a mother-child relationship*.

2. It has an α-element structure:

I postulate *an α-element version* of a private Oedipus myth which is the means, the pre-conception, by virtue of which the infant is able to establish contact with the parents as they exist in the world of reality. The mating of this α-element Oedipal pre-conception with the realization of the actual parents gives rise to the conception of parents.

(1963, p. 93; italics BN)

We can extend this description of the Oedipal pre-conception to all pre-conceptions. It can thus be understood as a *pre-configured relationing of α-elements*. I.e., the pre-conceptional α-elements are not sense impressions and sensations transformed by the α-function but exist before all experience, yet still require reality (realization) in order to become initialized and effective. The pre-conception must encounter a positive realization that sufficiently saturates the state of expectation. This saturation must take place through a realization that has an existence *independent* of the personality (see Bion, 1965, p. 137). If this is successful, a conception emerges, which we can now understand as the initialization of the pre-configured relationing of the α-elements, into which the raw sense impressions transformed into α-elements are integrated.

In the relational dynamic between mother and child, or analyst and analysand, an asymmetry comes into play: the projected sense impressions, preconceptually interwoven and directed, enable the mother to sense the non-sensory dimension and to expect her child in his state. With realization (T→O), the mother-child relationship is then there to become present (O→K) in sublation. I have tried to describe this event as a moment of presence.

The real psychic in the moment of presence

In the presence moment, two pre-conceptions, namely that of the child and that of the mother, and different arousal and sensory impressions meet. In the presence moment, the two dimensions that are not sensual (and can only be intuited on this side and beyond the moment), namely the pre-conception and the experienced state, then show themselves. The pre-conception is realized and its α-structure is initialized: The child is there, the mother is there, the relationship is there. At the same time, the experienced state itself is there without sensual quality. It will become apparent afterwards ("nachträglich") what it will have been. This is an extremely condensed, circular-paradoxical moment, which is nevertheless of the greatest clarity and unambiguity. The previous considerations make it more understandable. The paradox-circular, non-sensory complexity can only be grasped by pure perceptual consciousness, as described above. The reflexive ego, which is attached to the secondary process and the reality principle, is absent.

Let us stay with the example of the child being afraid of dying. The child has the sensual bare experience, cries it out, but this cry is addressed by the pre-conception to the expected breast. The mother, deeply lovingly oriented toward her child (her pre-conception) therefore hears this cry as a call. She takes her infant in her arms, mother, child and relationship are there, a positive realization. The α-structure of the pre-conception → conception is initialized and the anxiety, i.e. the state itself, is now really there. At the same time, time and space are there, from which the times past, present and future become and the three-dimensional space emerges. This moment of presence occurs in pure "limited consciousness".

For me, very fundamental questions arise at this point: What is the psychic? If we stay in the example: Is it the fear (of dying) that shows itself in the relationship in time and space? Or is it the fear in the relationship in time and space? In the first case, the real psychic would be "anxiety itself", in the second case, anxiety and the realized pre-conception and time and space. So in the second case, anxiety itself would only be a component of the real psychic, which still includes the initialized relationship (and time and space).

This question sounds very epistemologically academic. But it is not. For we must ask whether anxiety is really qualityless. This brings us to the questions that already played a role in the Freud-Klein controversy. For Fechner, von Helmholz, and thus for Freud (but also for modern thinkers like Maturana), qualities must emerge from impulses. Transposed to our example, the question arises: does anxiety show up in the moment of presence as fear of dying or must it be created by the actors (mother-child; analyst-analysand) in $O \rightarrow K$?

Clinical example: Moment of presence

I would like to discuss this question briefly using the opening example (see Nissen, 2013).

The beginning of the analysis of Mrs. A. was surprisingly lively. When I leave my office to go to the practice I have to walk along a small garden path so that patients who arrive early (as Mrs. A. always did) can see me coming. When she saw me coming, she was like a small child who sees her mother, excitedly waving her arms and kicking her legs. Although there was no motor discharge of this kind, her eyes were shining and I had a feeling of deep joy inside me. The treatment was a friendly get-together: we had a similar sense of humor, we liked the same things, and the patient was well aware of this. But the nameless dimensions were not absent, a juxtaposition of a lively sensual world with non-existence arose, and the two do not seem to touch each other. From this tension between elated bliss and nothingness, minute attunements developed between the patient and me. The nameless was present as a negative. Diffuse, dark, almost physically sensual, trace elements of the nameless gathered and worked in situ in me.

Parallel to my condensed presentiments a change occurred in the patient. After approximately seven to eight months of treatment, the patient began to avert her gaze when I arrived. She gave me a little smile, lowered her gaze or looked away. I was irritated. At the same time she appeared in her accounts of her anonymous sexual practices and depictions of loneliness as an uninvolved, uncomprehending observer, as if asking: "Why do they do that?" Her visits to the toilet were described in detail: frequency, consistency, pain, and her fears of chronic diseases.

At this time there was a tension in the air which is difficult to describe, an apprehension and fear of a realization which, at last, culminated in a touch. Instead of sitting on the chair and waiting, the patient had gone to the toilet. When greeting me, she hesitated to shake hands. Her hands were still damp. She was silent. She then said she had wondered about shaking my hand as before the session at home she had had her feces in her hands. She had washed her hands thoroughly, also using disinfectant, but felt she had to wash her hands again here. For the first time I felt a moment of disgust and inner dissociation. I said she was afraid of touching me and contaminating me with this issue, but she also wished that it would at last find its place in the analysis.

After approximately one year, the nameless contents spilled into a session. The patient indicated that she had once again practiced "it" by herself in the bath. In a moment of presence the scene existed for the patient and for me. A discovery of the psychic itself, the nameless state, the patient, myself, and the relationship. For a moment a forlorn nothingness was there, which could be best paraphrased as getting lost in a dark, dumb, infinite space.

Many psychic qualities surfaced in O→K: I knew how she felt: lonely and ceasing to be; I knew what the atmosphere was: icy and cold, where only the warmth of her feces remained; I knew how the feces tasted: inflammatory, even though this is not exactly a taste, and so on. I no longer remember the exact words of my interpretation, but I told her the central emotional qualities and added the following words: "You're going to die this way".

Back to our question: How does the psychic itself, the real psychic, show itself in the moment of presence? Does the forlorn nothingness with its qualities show up in the presence moment or does the nonentity show up and the "secondary" qualities are determined in the O→K transformation? Both are possible, but I believe that the presence moment is without any quality. Just as the mother with her faculty can predetermine qualities in her baby's cry and thus hear the cry as a call, pre-conceptual and qualitative presentiments developed in me in advance to the presence moment: I forebode the crushing danger the patient was in and my responsibility—hence I could say, "You're going to die this way". At the same time, in my reverie, I "dreamt" the patient's communications of her anonymous sex and practices, experienced the moist, cool hands, and the loneliness and fear in the patient's voice, gaze, and expression had an almost physical effect on me. So I heard a kind of call from her, to which I could then give words, names, after the moment of presence.

In the moment of presence, the relationship and the nothingness (Nichtung) in time and space have become real and irrefutable. The sensual phenomena in the antecedent—pre-qualified by the capacity of the object—are in the moment of presence, which is paradoxically completely without quality, and are defined in the transformation to K.

The sublation of the moment of presence in conception and in thought

The object must be able to psychically qualify the antecedent phenomena—realized in the moment of presence in the relationship—in such a way that they sublate the experience (in the sense of Hegel). If the presentative word presentations deviate too much from experience, misconceptions arise (see Bion, e.g. 1965, p. 137; see also Freud's word presentation and thing presentation).

The presence moment pushes toward sublation. To my knowledge, this process has not yet been clarified (see Nissen, 2015). Bion remarks: "a relevant constellation will be evoked during the process of at-one-ment with O, the process denoted by transformation O→K" (1970, p. 33). The term "constellation" represents "the process precipitating a constant conjunction" (1970, p. 33, footnote 1). Why will a relevant constellation be evoked? A difficult question to answer. I had speculated in 2015 that time enforces it, but now think it might be the reflexive consciousness, which can only be temporarily suspended. When it comes back into its own, the moment of presence is submerged.

Freud conceived of (reflexive) consciousness as a sense organ for perceiving psychic qualities (see Freud, 1900, p. 615; Bion refers to this formulation several times, for example in 1962a). With the derivation, this formulation becomes more comprehensible: in the moment of presence, there can only be the perceptual consciousness that grasps the real psychic. Bion writes: "its (O - BN) presence can be recognized and felt, but it cannot be known" (1970, p. 30). The qualification of sensory experience is then undertaken by reflexive consciousness, recalling the perceived secondary qualities. The relationship, the realized pre-conception, and the α-elementary qualification of the state thus yield the psychic, which now has a name. In the name is the relationship, even if it refers to the secondarily qualified state. The interpretation of the mother, "Are you so scared (of dying)", is the recognition of the relationship, is the relationship with the mother as a present and absent object. This interpretation is a sublation of the moment of presence into the presentative. I borrow the term presentational symbol from Susan Langer (1942). It captures a state that is so complex that it can only be preserved in the presentative symbol, never fully described discursively.

This shows that every interpretation is a sublation and includes three facets: we *discover* states, i.e. structures and dynamics, in the analysand asymmetrically in the relationship—and establish the relationship. At the same time, however, what is discovered is a *creation* of the analytic couple. What is discovered shows itself in the moment of presence, and yet will have been created by the couple. With the sublation into the presentative, the created discovered is then determined, whereby this determination is beyond the sovereignty of the participants, *subjugating* them in an overpowering way (see also Ogden, 1994). Nevertheless, it must be empirically correct, i.e. it must be connectable. After all, the participants believe that they empirically share the same thing. Presentational symbolism with its vagueness makes a lot possible here, but it remains strictly speaking an erroneous belief—a reassuring erroneous belief.

In the example, these facets are revealed: the forlorn nothingness was discovered, the specific qualities (inflammatory taste as a condensation of eating feces and intestinal inflammation) were created in the process by the couple and the couple was "subjugated" by the force of the after-sentence ("you're going to die this way").

With the transformation to K, a conception has been created—and this in the *witnessing* of the object/analyst. This point is important; for the infant, as well as for patients struggling with nameless states, conception cannot outlast the absence of the object. For this it must become a thought.

The demand the infant (the analysand) is now faced with is that the developed preconception "breast" has to "mate" with the rejection, meaning that after the hallucinatory wish fulfilment it has to endure the "exigencies of life" (Freud, 1900, p. 564). From this mating a thought emerges: "if the capacity for toleration of frustration is sufficient the 'no-breast' inside becomes a thought, and an apparatus for 'thinking' it develops" (Bion, 1962b, p. 307). With the thought that the absent object is the same as that which was present, and with the thought that the absent is present in me, it can be recognized that the absent, needed, and also hated object is the same as the present, breastfeeding, and loved object. Bion already ascribes an experience of truth to this realization:

> a sense of truth is experienced if the view of an object which is hated can be conjoined to a view of the same object when it is loved, and the conjunction confirms that the object experienced by different emotions is the same object. A correlation is established.
>
> (1962b, p. 310)

But I cannot go into this complex process here (for more details, see Nissen, 2021a; see also Winnicott: "The Use of an Object", 1969).

Discovering the nameless

In many case studies of the nameless (or in autistoid, autistic states, those of breakdown etc.) the transference dynamics are determined by the experience of the analyst. It cannot be otherwise. For our Cs is the organ that can grasp the psychic life on the basis of communication from Ucs to Ucs. However, there is a massive complication in nameless dynamics: the failure of projective identification as the preferred communication mechanism of the psychic. As explained in the theoretical discussion, the grasping of the psychic is heavily dependent on the sensory phenomena being addressed objectally, so that the object can predetermine their qualities and the relationship can be experienced. If this dynamic fails, the object is hardly able to grasp states or can only try to imagine them in himself. Parents of autistic children repeatedly report that they have not been able to hear their child's cry as a call; people suffering from severe hypochondriacal anguish cannot communicate Ucs their anxiety, only complain that they are afraid of death because they have a fatal tumor. The hypochondriacal anxiety seems absurd, the nameless anxiety is not grasped (see Nissen, 2018). People with severe depression can no longer communicate their mental death and suicidal tendencies (see Nissen, 2016). Countless other examples could be listed; we now know how many symptoms conceal such dynamics (overview e.g. Nissen, 2008; Rhode, 2018). However, the immediate experience of those affected, often as nameless dread, usually remains hidden from us.

However, there are forms of coming into more direct contact with the psychic life of patients who have given up hope of a containing object and no longer communicate in a projective-identificatory way. Benedetti (1983) speaks here of osmosis, Moser (2021) of permeability, I have described it as an inductive process (e.g. Nissen, 2014 or 2021b). Although the patients do not address an object, we are "sucked in" to their experience. It is not an identification, not a symbiosis, and not a delusion—as Moser (2021) points out. It is an intense, overwhelming involvement in which the reflexive functions of consciousness and reality-oriented sides of the ego are almost forcibly suspended and we stagger helplessly and will-lessly into the world of the patient. We become the patient's experience, there is no longer any question of communication from Ucs to Ucs. Thus the functions we need to grasp and digest projective identifications are suspended, e.g. the α-function. The difference with becoming O might be that Faith (F) is absent (see Bion, 1970).

I would now like to circle the nameless in such experiences in analysis and begin with a short example of an inductive process (see Nissen, 2021b). The patient, Mrs. B., has experienced severe and continuous traumatization. I try to reproduce some moments of this dissolution. They are fragments, reduced by me to a few sentences, much more confused in the situation, encompassing many minutes.

I was with Max, suddenly he was standing in the room, we were wearing clothes, the child had, I had something with him once, sex, was it sex? 15 years ago, all full of rubbish. How did Ludwig get into the room? Crazy, huh? Sarah never came, not even in the evening. It was a party, really loud. There was nothing going on with Sarah, but she wants to give me her jacket. It's damaged, in the bin. W. (first name of an internationally known artist) was drunk, I've known him forever, with bottle. Sarah's in bed, at her party, can you imagine? Probably with Keith...

While the patient—much more confused and disoriented in the scene—is talking, she lies as if in shock, with a slight head tremor, while making defensive movements with one hand.

I will now first write what I knew about the material at this point:

Max is an older man with whom she fell a little in love. Ludwig was probably standing in the room where she was lying with Max, still dressed. Did Ludwig have a child in his arms? Ludwig is 75 years old, did she have sex with him 15 years ago? She wasn't even 10 years old then! Sarah, depressive acquaintance of her mother's age, probably had a party, was lying in bed (or is she still lying in bed?). Sarah once gave the patient a jacket, which she threw away, always afraid it would be discovered. The patient's father worked with W. at times. Keith's been dead for five years.

But I no longer had this knowledge at my disposal. For I was infected by the dissolution of thinking. A panic arose in me, I would go crazy, psychotic, if I continued to listen. This is not a paraphrase of a feeling or a counter-transference, but a real fear, panic, from which I wanted to flee inwardly. I wanted to get out of my body, felt helpless, at the mercy, panicked that this was not possible. I know all kinds of reactions to similar material (depersonalizing, distancing, e.g. taking refuge in rationalizing, etc.). But in this scene the threateningness was different: a being at the mercy and a panic threat that it would really happen, happen unavoidably.

For the patient, it was no message to the analyst, no communication, a fortiori no psychic communication—and yet this event is of extraordinary importance. With this being infected, I knew about the dissolution, I felt the being pulled into the maelstrom of dissolution in my own body, felt the hopeless horror. So this scene changed the encounter between us. If I spoke of dissolution, disintegration etc. after this experience, the patient hears that someone is speaking who has experienced something, knows something about it. Understanding as *holding* and *preparation* for sublation.

This scene does not represent a moment of presence, is not O. Neither was the experience in the relationship—everyone was on their own and had to "save" themselves, "survive" the scene. Also, sensual qualities dominated this scene (see also Bion: "K, L, or H are inappropriate to O", 1965, p. 140); it was so full of sensual overflow that it was almost unbearable—I wanted to get out of my body. It is also significant how I "saved" myself. I was unable to give any interpretation; such thinking, psychoanalytical faculty had been torn away. I was saved by a hint of reality. I said, "Keith is dead after all, died of drugs". She was silent, but somehow more grounded. So I regained my composure and was able to say, "Something is pressing on you, threatening you, making you lose yourself".

But this intervention does not establish a moment of presence; it prepares container/contained structures (see Bion, 1970, p. 27f). A presence moment requires the sublation into the presentative. Without this naming, the presence moment will not have been psychic, indeed in the worst case it can become retraumatizing. The moment of presence is relationship in which psychic quality shows itself. I have reintroduced reality in the example, thus contributing to a grounding of analyst and analysand. As I said before, I assume that in this unpredictable inductive process Faith was completely absent. Perhaps this loss corresponds to the abandonment of hope for a containing object in Mrs. B.'s previous life?

A few weeks after this scene, the treatment changed. Firstly, I began to discover a form of second skin that I had suspected but was blinded by the fascination of:

Mrs. B. had grown up under the most severe and pervasive traumatic conditions. She lived in the feeling of having to survive "physically" (as the patient herself put it) under these conditions and developed a sensual ability to grasp the inner worlds of others at lightning speed. She used the experience that often occurs in traumatic events, namely that everything is there in the greatest clarity and precision as time slows down. She distilled from this traumatic experience the ability to grasp the inner constellations and motives in the object at lightning speed and thus to orientate herself in the world that is psychically completely foreign to her. This ability took the form of a second-skin defense. I.e., she instantly perceives all inner and outer stirrings, impulses, and motives of the other person and thus grasps the inner world, primarily the primary-process dynamics, so precisely that she knows in a flash about the inner world of the other person. I once spoke of X-ray eyes for the innermost part of another. Since she is very clever and linguistically highly gifted, so has brilliant forms of expression, it seems as if it is a highly developed understanding of the psychic. But it is not an understanding of psychic structures and dynamics, but merely an inferential registering of phenomena that have no psychic quality. It was her way of surviving the traumatic world of her childhood.

The patient uses this ability to grasp the inner world of another like an X-ray to transform herself into the inner world of the object: she becomes so perfectly one with the object in thinking, feeling, assessment, humor, etc., that a feeling of consubstantiality, even unity of being, arises. She senses the other person's attitudes and perspectives on the world, and then expresses them in an extremely clever, skillful, and linguistically brilliant way, so that I kept thinking: "that's exactly how I see it too", "that's exactly what I think and feel! I couldn't express it better! How can she know that?" She would then sometimes ask: "Is that how you see it too?", which I would then sometimes confirm, still totally amazed. "Yes, really? That's crazy!" she would say. But some time after I was torn into her world of dissolution, a small irritation arose that led to the discovery: it wasn't the correspondence in content that she found "crazy", but that she had managed to get herself so turned on.

Then there was another suspicion: here and there I discovered that she absorbed my formulations, ideas, images or reflections and immediately used them in her artistic work. Some time later, when she summarized something she had written, my formulations or images or the like appeared one-to-one. Whether she was aware of it, I don't know. But this discovery also created a new, more separate positioning toward her. I got to see her.

The clever patient, who seismographically registered tiny changes, felt this change. She had turned the analyst into an autistic object (Tustin, 1980) which was supposed to protect her from the perception of the not-self. Her two-dimensional second-skin world (see Bick, 1968; Meltzer, 1975a, b) was cracking, but self and object were not yet conceivable. What this form of namelessness in experience meant then became clear to me:

The patient reported a conflict with a dog owner at the end of a session. I had thoughtlessly and spontaneously made a remark that many dog owners are nuts (the patient knows that I have a dog). The patient was totally distraught, and asked stuttering, panic-stricken, confused, frozen: "Why?"

I reply, "Now I am another for you, there is a difference between us that confuses you". The patient replies totally confused, "No, no, not at all".

I now introduce the next session, which shows the birth of a separate object relationship, but one which does not yet exist:

MRS. B.: (already starting while lying down): "I was wondering why you think that dog owners are nuts. Thought it must have something to do with your environment. It's not like that where I am". (In a wooded area near my house there is a dog walking area with many neurotic dog owners, i.e. the patient is trying to justify the disturbance between us with this social situation).

PA: "The difference between us concerns you. You are discovering that I'm another. Am I nuts?"

MRS. B.: "Yes, no, but I don't understand. Maybe because this is the exercise area. There the dogs are in stress, owners then too or something".

PA: (I feel that the fact that I'm another is confusing her): "Mhm."

MRS. B.: "I had a puppy a few years ago, I took it to a dog play area. As soon as I was in the meadow, all the dogs, a whole pack, came running down the hill toward him. It panicked. It screamed rhythmically, very cruelly (she *screams cruelly* too). It ran through a hole in the fence onto the road, two lorries had to brake hard and ran over it anyway, but it didn't get hurt."

PA: "What a panic, what a threat!"

MRS. B.: "Yes. Total shock for me..."

PA: "You seem shocked now, today too"

MRS. B.: "The other dog owners said they don't do anything. Is that true? Has anything like this ever happened to your dog?"

(Patient speaks threateningly and testingly.)PA: (hesitating): "Yes, that's how I know that something like that can be dangerous."

MRS. B.: "Thank God you say that. I know with wolves looking for a new pack, it's totally dangerous."

PA: "But maybe discovering that we can think different things is dangerous too."

MRS. B.: "What? No. (… missing something) Do you know X (well-known artist), a total boozer. He used to have a German Shepherd. So that he (the dog BN) didn't get bored, he bought him a sheep, which he then ran around in the garden for 14 days until the sheep dropped dead from stress."

PA: (She says it so funny that I have to smile a little [audibly]—she laughs too) "It's not funny in itself."

MRS. B.: "Nah, anyway, there are freaks like that. Are there freaks here too, there was something like that: 'Attention free-range pig' in the garden…"

PA: (a throbbing despair, hardly bearable, at the same time a kind of test again like with the dog/wolf pack): "That's right, we talked about that before, there was once a vet here who took in a three-legged wild boar, it lived with him in the garden and was called Schnitzel."

MRS. B.: (Laughs, relaxes) "I remember that right. That's funny. Really? That's a good name! There's a dog in my new book who also only has three legs."

(My sense is that she has just decided this and will take it on. I mean, I can feel how she always adapts immediately and takes over the same thing, negating differences like that. I have had this suspicion for some time, but this time it touches me unpleasantly.)

MRS. B.: "It's about a defense lawyer who only realizes at the trial who she is defending, a real cold-blooded sadist who bestially slaughters women. She decides to serve justice."

(Again extreme tension, even naked violence in the room. Silence in which every movement is disturbing, every sound would become a treacherous noise. In the session, for the first time, there is a kind of transference, but which one? I don't dare address them. Who is lawyer, who is murderer? Who is perpetrator, who is victim? It is so confused that nothing can be distinguished. I get indescribably scared, and think I shouldn't have started the treatment.)

MRS. B.: "As she continues the defense, she becomes responsible for another murder."

PA: (after a short pause): "Who is the other? What do you do when you realize the truth, that is, see what is real? Does it become murderous or can it be endured?"

MRS. B.: "Yes. (Pause) Was just thinking of Kant, it's all about truth, then you were talking about truth."

PA: (Again, an adjustment. I am rather defensive, since Kant is not about truth, but about the limits of knowledge. The adaptations don't putty over the differences but tear them open further. Fear and aversive feelings again! I catch myself, but the session is almost over. I think, saying something now can be too much, but saying nothing is not possible.) Then I say something like: "I think we have to see that something has happened between us. How dangerous is that?"

MRS. B.: (barely audible) "mhm." Then "hmm".

This session sounds quite harmless, but it is not. I had never before experienced such naked, nameless horror with such intensity. There was really nothing to distinguish, nothing to make out: who am I, who is she; who is crazy, is nuts; who is the murderer, who is being bestially slaughtered, who is pack, who is pup, who is circling who here, who is stressed to the point of death. Who discovers, who is lawyer, who is accused. Is continuation of treatment/ mandate fatal? If I violently bite my own arm, do I eat or am I eaten? Total confusion. The violence is so concrete that I don't know for sure if something is or isn't happening. I have the feeling that I can't interpret anything: I can't find a name for this murderous violence, for the confusion, for the parasitic appropriation. Nor is the relationship there. Who is who? Am I another? I am hardly able to discern a self-object relationship, however partial and momentary. Is the discovery of self and object an annihilation? That is why I do not dare (or am not able) to interpret in the relationship: interpretation is relationship (sic!), is separateness/separation, is punctuation that could lead to murder or to being torn off (see Tustin, 1980, 1988). Is the continuation of the treatment fatal?

The naming of annihilation is only possible in relationship, but in annihilation there is no relationship. An aporetic paradox. But this form of inductive experience makes recognition possible: I suffer such states also (see Bion, 1970, p. 9). The hope arises of being able to discover it.

At the same time, I think it is very important to see the progression in this dynamic: it is an approach to the facticity of separateness (one of the facts of life): separateness is being torn off, annihilation, extinction *and* being born, coming into the world, being recognized and held, being in a secure place. Both are there at the same time. It is hard to think: we are drawn to linear-serial, logical thinking, but it is aporetic, parallel-circular, paradoxical.

Mrs B. is working on exactly that. She wants to know what is true, what is real. She senses that she needs "truth" and "reality"—only then will she be able to be psychic. There is a desire for truth; so twice she tests me (pack; vet). Here she must have an objectal dimension. She asks: "Who are you? Are you being honest with me? If you are another, are you annihilating or giving life?" Also, that she tries to release the unbearable tension in anecdotes is not only defense against relationship but also perception of relationship. Something in her is trying to regulate a tension in the relationship.

I try not to "go down" in the session and I try to approach, to prepare for the discovery of separateness to appear and communicate that it will be a catastrophic change with a truly unpredictable outcome. Faith (F) was attacked. What has helped is the experience of nameless states unfolding in such a way as to create container-contained structures.

Concluding remarks

In the clinical examples, nameless states show up in different forms: in the opening example, Mrs A., everything is spoken and described quite clearly, but nothing is suffered and discovered. On the contrary, the words, which contain nothing psychic, rather disguise the nameless threat.

The state of dissolution that I experience with Mrs B., on the other hand, lets me experience the disintegration in somatoform, sensual violence. The reflexive ego threatens to disappear, I try to survive, whereby the "I" gets caught up in the whirlpool of dissolution. It would be more precise to say that a living being, an organism, is trying to save itself. It is a relationshipless state in which each organism (analyst & analysand) fights for itself, even the holding function seems absent. Thus no moment of presence, no O can occur. Subsequently, however, it is possible to capture the experience. This gives the sense data a predetermination and relates it to the patient and the relationship. In this way, this experience can be led back into holding and contribute to container-contained structures. Thus, a pre-conception arises in which the hope germinates that states that were not contained in her previous life experiences could still be containable—but without any guarantee!

Mrs B. could perceive very precisely that I had suffered something of the dissolution. But this also laid the nucleus that the analyst was another. The thesis was that pre-conceptions have α-element structure and are objectal. It is interesting that Mrs A., with her looking away and her wet hands, also enacted this objectal dimension in the run-up to O. In the case of Mrs B., who had already sensed the otherness with her seismographic feeling, the appearance of separateness then broke in with all its force. The whole decomposition of thinking, feeling, and acting took place. A nameless dynamic, not knowing whether one would be torn down, pushed into the black hole, eating or eaten oneself. This dynamic seems to me to be the mirror image of Mrs. B.'s past, in which the child gave up hope of a containing object. We can thus grasp something of the risk that our patients trustingly take—what an achievement!

When it then comes to a moment of presence, practically everything comes into being: the self, the object, the relationship, the times, the places. Mrs A. practiced a perversion in which her early experience was permanently repeated: feeding herself with excrement that she produced herself, smearing herself with excrement and urine and giving herself hold, completely lost, threatened by nothingness. In the moment of presence, completely without quality, this forlorn nothingness showed itself in the relationship. Thus it was "there" and could become in T→O. The presentational interpretation took up the secondary qualities that had probably shown up in the holding. With this, the real psychic was sublated. At the same time, the perversion practiced became "real", and for the first time the patient understood what she was doing for herself alone in the bathtub. With the psychic quality "inflamed taste" she realized, for example, that she was really eating her inflamed feces. She could see herself in the bathtub and knew that the analyst saw her doing it too. The perversion got a place and the times emerged: in the past she ate her feces, it is there in the present and will not be in the future (she gave up manifest perversion after the session!).

With this derivation, the treatment advice becomes more understandable that holding is so important in these processes. We should have as much patience as our patients have courage.

Notes

1 This example was discussed in detail in Nissen (2013). I prefer to draw on previously published clinical material for reasons of privacy and confidentiality, in order to discuss it in the new context and from the new vertex.
2 For a detailed discussion of the theoretical and metatheoretical foundations, see Nissen, 2021a & b.
3 In "Learning from Experience", Bion drops the distinction between inner and outer world (chapter two, §1). Sense data of the self therefore means that the inner and outer sense impressions are registered by the consciousness of the self.
4 In my opinion, the term "emotion" is an unfortunate choice because in my view emotions are already qualified inner impressions and sensations.
5 In 1962a Bion speaks of β-elements as non-altered, undigested sense impressions. This means that the "raw data" are not yet β-elements but become so only when the α function cannot affect them. Grotstein (2007) considers β-elements to be secondary, also referring to the choice of Greek letters.
6 I think the pre-conception is a development of Freud's idea of "primal phantasy". Freud speaks of primal phantasies as "phylogenetically inherited schemata, which, like the categories of philosophy, are concerned with the business of 'placing' the impressions derived from actual experience.... Wherever experiences fail to fit in with the hereditary schema, they become remodelled in the imagination. ... We are often able to see the schema triumphing over the experience of the individual" (Freud, 1918, p. 119). A little later Freud writes: "it is hard to dismiss the view that some sort of hardly definable knowledge, something, as it were, preparatory to an understanding, was at work in the child at the time" (ibid., p. 120).

References

Benedetti, G. (1983). *Todeslandschaften der Seele.* Vandenhoeck & Ruprecht.
Bick, E. (1968). The experience of the skin in early object-relations. *Int J Psychoanal,* 49, 484–486.
Bion, W.R. (1962a). *Learning from experience.* Tavistock.

Bion, W.R. (1962b). The psycho-analytic study of thinking. *Int. J. Psycho-Anal.*, 43:306–310.

Bion, W.R. (1963). *Elements of psycho-analysis*. Heinemann.

Bion, W.R. (1965). *Transformations*. Heinemann.

Bion, W.R. (1970). *Attention and interpretation*. Tavistock.

Freud, S. (1900). The interpretation of dreams. In *S.E.* (Vol. 4). Hogarth.

Freud, S. (1915). The unconscious. In *S.E.* (Vol. 14). Hogarth.

Freud, S. (1918). From the history of an infantile neurosis. In *S.E.* (Vol. 17). Hogarth.

Grotstein, J.S. (2007). *A beam of intense darkness. Wilfred Bion's legacy to psychoanalysis.* Karnac Books.

Langer, S.K. (1942). *Philosophy in a new key.* Harvard University Press.

Meltzer D. (1975a). The psychology of autistic states and of post-autistic states. In D. Meltzer, J. Bremner, S. Hoxter, D. Weddell, & I. Wittenberg, *Explorations in autism* (pp. 6–29. Clunie.

Meltzer D. (1975b). Dimensionality in mental functioning. In D. Meltzer, J. Bremner, S. Hoxter, D. Weddell, & I. Wittenberg, *Explorations in autism* (pp. 223–239). Clunie.

Moser, U. (2021). Kommentar zu Bernd Nissen: Das Erleben von Auflösung. *Jahrbuch der Psychoanalyse*, 84, 223–226.

Nissen, B. (2008). On the determination of autistoid organizations in non autistic adults. *Int. J. Psycho-Anal.*, 89, 261–277.

Nissen, B. (2013). On mental elements. Based on the example of an autistoid perversion. *Int. J. Psycho-Anal.*, 94: 239–256.

Nissen, B. (2014). Autistoide Organisationen. *Jahrbuch der Psychoanalyse*, 68, 71–88.

Nissen, B. (2015). Faith (F) and presence moment (O) in analytic processes: An example of a narcissistic disorder. *Int. J. Psycho-Anal.*, 96, 1261–1281.

Nissen, B. (2016). Melancholie und Zusammenbruch. Eine Neubetrachtung von Freuds „Trauer und Melancholie". *Jahrbuch der Psychoanalyse*, 73, 123–146.

Nissen, B. (2018). Hypochondria as an actual neurosis. *Int. J. Psycho-Anal.*, 99, 103–124.

Nissen, B. (2021a). What is the psychic, how can it be grasped and understood? *The Scandinavian Psychoanalytic Review.* doi:10.1080/01062301.2021.1930505.

Nissen, B. (2021b). Das Erleben von Auflösung. *Jahrbuch der Psychoanalyse*, 84, 217–223.

Ogden, T.H. (1994). *Subjects of analysis.* Karnac Books.

Rhode, M. (2018). Object relations approaches to autism. *Int. J. Psycho-Anal.*, 99(3), 702–724.

Tustin, F. (1980). Autistic objects. *Int. Rev. Psycho-Anal.*, 7, 27–39.

Tustin, F. (1988). The 'black hole'. *Free Associations*, 1, 35–50.

Winnicott, D.W. (1969). The use of an object. *Int. J. Psycho-Anal.*, 50, 711–716.

Winnicott, D.W. (1974). Fear of breakdown. *Int. Rev. Psycho-Anal.*, 1, 103–107.

Chapter 3

To feel in my flesh[1]

Receptivity, resonance, and the beta screen

Howard B. Levine

I

It is difficult to imagine a moment in one's existence without it being accompanied and qualified by some kind of "experience". However, as the Symingtons note, following Bion, that "experience" is often ineffable and beyond the full description of our thought or words: "at the heart of the human creature lies a mystery of which all conceptualizations are inadequate representations" (Symington & Symington, 1996, p. 51). The kind of experience of interest to psychoanalysts is that of unconsciously influenced emotional experience and as Bion (1962) said, the latter "cannot be conceived of in isolation from a relationship" (p. 42).

Emotion implies affect. Affect is rooted in the soma and accompanied by and/or related to physical sensations. Taken together, these simple statements cannot help but lead to the conclusion that despite the fragmenting potential of various psychoanalytic theories—one-person vs. two-person, intrapsychic vs. interpersonal, or object relational, etc.—experience, emotion, relationship, psyche, and soma constitute an ensemble that is intimately and inextricably connected. Apparent connections and disconnections between these various elements will depend in part upon the observational perspective from which they are seen and the purposes for which they are being taken note of.

When seen from the vertex of everyday life and consensually validatable, "common sense" reality, the practice of psychoanalysis, with its attempt to address emotional experience, psychic reality, psychic development, and psychic functioning, may appear at times to be counter-intuitive, elusive, confusing, even arcane. As Bion (1962) noted, a particular "problem presented by psycho-analytic experience is the lack of any adequate terminology to describe it" (p. 68). In addition to problems that may arise from the unconscious or deliberate misuse of language (i.e., lying), this lack reflects the degree to which a specialized "language of psychoanalysis" has not yet been completely and successfully developed and articulated. Inevitably, we find ourselves up against the very limitations of language itself, where we are confronted with the challenge of trying to fully convey or describe something

DOI: 10.4324/9781003534365-3

about human life and emotional experience.[2]Bion (1970) indicated this problem when he asserted that "mental space [i.e., the human psyche] is a thing-in-itself, that is infinite and unknowable, but ... [nevertheless] can be represented by thoughts" (Bion, 1970, p. 11).[3]

There is a disparity—and a slippage—as one moves from the thing-in-itself, raw, existential Experience[4] (**O**), to what can be known of that experience (**K**) and again as that knowable part, what we colloquially call "experience" written with a small e, is spoken of and perhaps too, even as it is thought about.[5] That is, there is an inevitable difference between what is sensuously *felt* and what can be *known* as one moves from unknowable, raw, existential Experience (**O**) to what can be known of that experience (**K**). This limitation in *translation* [6] also occurs as one attempts to speak and put the knowable part of our perceptions and feelings into words. It is likely that there is a gradient or trajectory from raw existential Experience, to not-yet-articulated thought, to that portion of thought that can be verbalized in which, at each point of transition, an unknowable, untransformable residue remains left behind.[7] This formulation becomes especially relevant as we explore Bion's attempts to expand psychoanalytic theory so as to enable us to "approach a mental life unmapped by the theories elaborated for the understanding of neurosis" (Bion, 1970, p. 37).

In his introduction to *Attention and Interpretation*, Bion (1970) cautioned readers about the limits and inadequacy of "words and verbal formulations" (p. 1), the very things that patients and analysts are necessarily forced to resort to and rely upon: "reason is emotion's slave and exists to rationalize emotional experience. Sometimes the function of speech is to communicate experience to another; sometimes it is to miscommunicate experience to another" (p. 1).

Later in the book, when contrasting the practice of psychoanalysis to the practice of medicine, he notes that problems of communication in psycho-analysis also arise from the fact that direct access to or recognition of the fundamental elements of psychoanalytic concern, *emotions* and raw, existential *Experience*, cannot come to be known empirically via the physical senses:

> the physician is dependent on realization of sensuous experience in contrast with the psycho-analyst whose dependence is on experience that is not sensuous. The physician can see and touch and smell. The realizations with which a psycho-analyst deals cannot be seen or touched; anxiety has no shape or colour, smell or sound.
>
> (Bion, 1970, p. 7)

Bion (1970) believed that since words and verbal formulations "develop from a background of sensuous experience" (p. 1), they inevitably prove limited, even reductive, if used in an attempt to describe and to convey the non-sensuously derived objects that are relevant to psychoanalytic inquiry and study. His reasoning about the origins of words and verbal formulations was similar to that of Freud (1923), who argued that "word presentations" in the psyche were derived from the infant's experience of *hearing* the spoken word. "These word-presentations are residues of memories; they were at one time perceptions, and like all mnemic residues they can become conscious again" (p. 20).

In Bionian terms, we could perhaps say that in the process of the construction and acquisition of language, the infant uses the physical sound envelope of the spoken word as a container for the memory trace of an emotion and relational experience and that the linkage of these components then creates—or is in some way related to the creation of—the signifying, semantic meaning of the word as a marker of a constant conjunction and representation (symbol or signifier) related to a transaction with or emotion about or associated with an absent object. This sensuous grounding of language, while extremely useful for certain kinds of communication, especially that related to the inanimate world, renders the semantic, word-based communications of language only partially able to encompass, fully describe, and transmit information about the data of raw existential Experience, psychic reality, and emotional life.

For Bion, then, although discourse and language are fundamental to "the talking cure" and probably better than any of the alternatives, relying upon them means trying to make the best of a bad situation. "Talking ... must be considered as potentially two different activities, one as a mode of communicating thoughts and the other as an employment of *musculature* to disencumber the personality of thoughts" (Bion, 1962, p. 83).

In the latter instance, thoughts may be unconsciously felt or considered to be equivalent or analogous to concrete things, unwanted accretions of stimuli, both because of or independent of their content. The problems that result for psychoanalysts and their patients from all of these complexities and inadequacies of language is captured in the refrain repeated by the character in T.S. Eliot's (1963) poem, *Sweeney Agonistes*,

> It ain't no good, it ain't no good,
>
> I gotta use words when I talk to you.

II

The limitations of language confound our attempts to write or talk about psychoanalysis with each other. They can become even more problematic when we offer our patients interpretations of what we feel may be happening. How to face, know, and speak about—acknowledge, bear, and put into perspective—the disappointments, pains, and terrors of life is at the heart of the matter.

The need to connect to and communicate with others is fundamental to being human. In fact, Bergstein (2019) suggests that "the urge to communicate, alongside the difficulty in communicating, seems to be the Ariadne's thread running throughout Bion's work" (Bergstein, 2019, p. 98). This observation applies to the analyst as well as the patient. "Communicating" refers both to talking to another and trying to understand something for and often about one's self. In either case, talking or thinking may be:

- used to increase contact with reality, oneself, or another;
- be used as a means of avoiding the pain of ignorance and not knowing (rationalizations, falsehoods, and other evasions of truth);
- or be used as a form of evacuation intended "to unburden the psyche of accretions of stimuli" (Bion, 1962, pp. 28 & 31) (thereby denying or destroying contact with reality).[8]

Following Freud (1911), Bion (1962) wrote:

> In his paper on Two Principles of Mental Functioning, Freud says … 'Thought [which Freud suggested was developed from ideation for the purpose of restraining action] was endowed with qualities which made it possible for the mental apparatus to support increased tension during a delay in the process of discharge'.
>
> (p. 28)

If this delay is better attuned to the demands and restrictions of reality than the initial wish or desire, then any frustration implicit in the delay of gratification may be offset by the "safety" or rewards of an alternative—more reality oriented—gratification that could be substituted for the original desire.[9]

The potential conflict implied here, between the Pleasure Principle and the Reality Principle, is no small matter. For both Freud and Bion, the birth of thought and the capacity to think are dependent upon a degree of frustration caused by an absent, ungratifying object.[10] Keeping the stress of that frustration within optimal, tolerable limits is what proves crucial. Thoughts or their precursors, primitive proto-thoughts, are initiated by the experience of *something* (environmental provision) that is needed but felt to be absent. Bion (1962) argues that these sequelae are apt to be felt as if they were "bad, needed objects" that must be gotten rid of

> because they are bad. They can be gotten rid of either by evacuation or modification. The problem is solved by evacuation if the personality is dominated by the impulse to evade frustration and by thinking the

objects if the personality is dominated by the impulse to modify the frustration.

(p. 84)

This explanation has relevance for our understanding of the question of mind-body integration.[11] From an economic point of view, if thought is an alternative to discharge-in-action as a way of relieving the psyche of an unwanted accretion of painful or potentially disequilibrating stimuli, then psyche may be seen as a physically rooted component of a somato-psychic *system*. From this perspective, the commonly assumed Cartesian split between mind and body dissolves, as thought and the process of thinking reveal their deep roots in the physicality of somatic tension regulation.[12]

The indissoluble interrelationship between mind and body, mind as rooted in and a component of the body, is also seen in Bion's (1962) assertion that the process of "coming to know", the **K** link, *is an emotional experience* (p. 47). Emotions and their derivatives are not only psychic events, but have a quality that is experienced physically, sensually and are often unconsciously co-determined by the actual qualities of the Other with whom the self, infant, patient, or analyst is in relation.

As Abel-Hirsch (2019) reminds us: "we are more used to conceiving of the mind/body relation in terms of the representation of the body in the mind. Bion [in *Memoir of the Future*, 1991] has the body speak its own language" (p. 568).

Can we then say that the mind "feels" and the "body speaks" in the feeling tone that appears to accompany and give credence and power to what we come to recognize (*feel*) as true?

To summarize, Bion argued, as did Freud, that thought, and/or the capacity to think thoughts, originates in reaction to an object's failure to respond in some needed way, provided that the consequences of that failure, which can take various forms such as absence, mis-attunement, non-receptivity, reversed projective identification, etc., can be kept within tolerable limits. But if that frustration or absence exceeds whatever the individual's level is of "tolerable", then the result will be measures designed to evade frustration rather than recognize, think about, and modify it. The important lesson for the treatment situation is this: "the choice that matters to the psycho-analyst is one that lies between procedures designed to evade frustration and those designed to modify it. That is the critical decision" (Bion, 1962, p. 29, original italics).

III

Bion (e.g., 1970) often said that humans need truth for psychic growth and well-being the way that the body needs alimentation. His formulations of the communicative aspect of projective identification and theory of alpha function and container/contained imply that the receptivity, resonance, and psychic processing capacity (alpha function) of an object may be necessary to the self's maintenance of the optimal degree of psychic tension needed for self-stabilization and psychic growth. This unconscious, dyadic, inter-subjective pairing is something that Bion implicitly linked to the determination and acquisition of truth.

Patients, especially non-neurotic (borderline and psychotic) patients, who tend toward avoidance of psychic reality and evacuation of emotional truth, may require the analyst's alpha function and interpretations to help them self-regulate, tolerate affects associated with self-knowledge (truth), and bridge the gap between representation and realization (Bion, 1970, p. 9).[13]

In pragmatic terms, this often means helping patients to notice, name, understand, and attend to what they are unable to contain and metabolize. It is the uncontainable, unknowable, ineffable storms of emotion and/or proto-emotion that cause or threaten to cause great anguish and terror that are at the center of what so many patients—and sometimes analysts—are trying to rid themselves of. This requirement becomes intensified and more urgent, when the analyst is faced with a psychotic patient or attempts to engage with what has become known as the psychotic part of the neurotic patient's personality or that part of their own.[14]

As his theory evolved, Bion's (1970) description of the object's participation in this process increasingly moved beyond that of naming, interpreting, and re-presenting—all activities in **K**—and spoke of the analyst's *being* and *becoming*—that is, *participation* in a process of *at-one-ment* and *becoming* the **O** of the patient.[15] However, he continued to characterize the analyst's interventions as "interpretations" even though their impact, meaning, and purpose may have been more as indicators of having reached a level of emotional contact, receptivity, resonance, and participation that was beyond—or perhaps before—their semantic content, rather than the understanding that that semantic content might imply.

While this level of participation is quite difficult to describe in words, it does indicate our need to take into consideration a dimension of the analyst's *being* rather than just "talking about", when thinking about the analyst's contribution to the homeostatic, psychic developmental movements mobilized in the analytic process. At any moment in that process, what will be decisive as to how or to what purposes thought or speech are assumed to be put—adaptation/sublimation or evacuation—will be the degree to which a given individual, patient, or analyst, at a given moment can accept not knowing (*negative capability*) and tolerate frustration. For Bion (1965, 1970), as for Winnicott (1960) in his famous pronouncement that there is no such thing as an infant, the extent and limits of frustration tolerance are often seen as determined by an unconscious, two-person, intersubjective process (container/contained). This is especially so in relation to the psychic development of the infant and child and in fostering psychic growth in the analytic situation.

It is the object's *receptivity* (the acceptance and/or formation of a *link*) that may prove decisive in allowing the patient to make contact through which the infant or patient's projective identifications (often of "bad", painful, or incomprehensible feelings and sensations) can be absorbed and allowed to dwell within the object, *resonated* with, and therein be subjected to *reverie* and the object's alpha function (i.e., transformed and metabolized) before being returned to the infant or patient in a more tolerable and/or comprehensible form.

An example of this appears in the conclusion to his paper *On Arrogance*, where Bion (1957) describes how his seemingly attacking and defensively projecting patient came to

> profit by ... the opportunity to split off parts of his psyche and project them into me ... and leave them there long enough for them to be modified by their sojourn in my psyche.... Associated with these experiences was a sense of being in contact with me, which I am inclined to believe is a primitive form of communication that provides a foundation on which, ultimately, verbal communication depends.
>
> (p. 92)

These are statements about the analyst's receptivity and non-receptivity to the patient's projective identifications and of the *necessity* of the analyst's allowing his or her self—included in its physically sensate dimension (i.e., somatic countertransference)—to be penetrated by those projections as a form of contact and communication, as well as the beginning steps in an intersubjective process of transformation. In regard to the latter, Symington and Symington (1996) suggest that beta elements, which by definition are not parts of thought and among which Bion (1962) included emotions, can have a sort of proto-consciousness and may be seen as possessing or evoking "an awareness of a lack of existence that demands an existence" perhaps in "a psyche seeking for a physical habitation to give it existence" (p. 121).

What may be confusing for some analysts is that these last comments offer a more positive view of these processes than has sometimes been assumed, even perhaps by Bion himself. At times, he seems to have been speaking of the motivation or underlying condition related to the projection, not as a cry for help or attempt at restitution, but as an attack or defense.[16] For example, in connection to his discussion of the beta-screen in *Learning from Experience*, he talks about patients who are unable to understand their own state of mind even when it is pointed out to them. These patients may be "saying words" but their "use of words is much closer to action intended to 'unburden the psyche of accretions of stimuli' than to speech" (Bion, 1962, p. 24).

This seems to continue a line of reasoning presented earlier in *Attacks on Linking*. There, Bion (1959) described how in some patients "the conduct of emotional life ... becomes intolerable. Feelings of hatred are thereupon directed against all emotions including hate itself, and against external reality, which stimulates them" (p. 107).

In his supervisions, Bion (Junqueiros et al., 2017) spoke of the possibility that the patient would stimulate memory or desire in the analyst as an attack or defensive maneuver meant to lead the analyst off course and indicated that following that pathway would only lead to futility. In *Cogitations*, reflecting on one such instance, he wrote:

> I am forced to have an emotional experience, and that I have to have it in such a way that I am unable to learn from it. I have consciousness, a sense organ enabling me to perceive the psychical qualities (as Freud puts it in *The Interpretation of Dreams*), but I am not to be allowed to comprehend it. Then I cannot learn by the emotional experience, and I cannot remember it.
>
> (Bion, 1992, p. 220)

With this in mind, Symington and Symington (1996) have said:

> The *beta screen* elicits feelings in the analyst rather than thinking which might eventuate in an interpretation, which in turn might get the patient in touch with the reality he hates and fears.... It is as though the function of the *beta screen* is to stop the analyst from thinking and instead to act out.
>
> (p. 66)

This is the usual interpretation. But let us look more closely at what Bion (1962) said when he defined the beta-screen:

> Thanks to the beta-screen the psychotic patient has a capacity for *evoking emotions* in the analyst; his associations are the elements of the beta-screen intended to evoke interpretations or other responses which are less related to his need for psycho-analytic interpretation than to *his need to produce an emotional involvement*.
>
> (p. 24, italics added)

Bion continues in a footnote (pp. 100–101) saying that the existence of the patient's "choice" to evoke feelings in and produce an emotional involvement with the analyst suggests the presence of *intuition* in the patient and implies unconscious purpose and intention controlled by the non-psychotic part of the personality. The "purpose" referred to seems to be in the service of survival: a *need to make contact by evoking feelings and an emotional involvement with the object*, because "the patient is starved of genuine therapeutic material, namely truth, and therefore ... his impulses that are directed to survival are overworked attempting to extract cure from therapeutically poor material" (Bion, 1962, footnote 10.1.1., pp. 100–101). And, perhaps, from an unreceptive, at the moment, therapeutically misguided analyst?

Could we not also see the analyst's (hopefully) momentary lack of receptivity and mis-attunement as a kind of role-responsiveness (Sandler, 1976), the result of having "successfully" unconsciously absorbed and actualized in a micro-traumatizing fashion the patient's unconscious projection of a problematic object relationship? This takes us back to Freud's (1912) assertion about the inevitability and even necessity of arousing actual moments of negative transference, because one cannot slay the enemy in absentia or in effigy (p. 108).

Returning to *On Arrogance*, we notice that while Bion (1957) began by describing the defensive arrogance of his patient, he wound up recognizing his own obstructive interference. He tells us that he ultimately recognized that his insistence on the "employment of verbal communication was felt by the patient to be a mutilating attack on … [the patient's] methods of communication" (p. 91).

If we view the patient's motivations from a communicative instead of a defensive or aggressive vertex and take what Bion says about the beta screen literally, we then might see the patient's activities as unconsciously offering the analyst a course correction. To what extent is the patient unconsciously trying to recruit the analyst into having an emotional experience in order to correct for a deficient or misguided emotional involvement on the analyst's part? Or to communicate and perhaps actualize through repetition a very negative emotional experience of incomprehension or tendency to discharge tension via action (acting out) rather than thought?

This sounds like Bion is describing an activation of the patient's survival instinct in the face of feeling overwhelmed or deprived of emotional contact.[17] It is as if in this way the patient is unconsciously saying:

> I don't feel us in contact and am trying to force a connection. I can't find or use words and so can't tell you what this is I am feeling or (unsuccessfully) struggling to contain and transform, and so I am inducing something in you that perhaps you can make sense of for/with me.

This matter of *evocation* may reflect the absence of emotional contact and the fact that the analyst's participation, receptivity, and permeability are required, perhaps as a precondition for the patient's ability to subsequently use the semantic meaning of an interpretation. This alternative perspective adds to the complexity of the clinical situation and suggests that factually "correct" interpretations without the necessary accompanying form of emotional involvement may be analytically ineffective.

IV

As Bion's theory evolved, the principal agent in the analytic process was increasingly described in terms of not necessarily coming to *know* that which was already formed but hidden in one's self (i.e., the repressed unconscious), but of facing or tolerating a truth about oneself or one's life situation, creating a functional life narrative—even a necessarily incomplete narrative—and developing the capacity to tolerate the distress of frustration and pain of knowing and not knowing (negative capability).

An essential component in this process entails the analyst's coming to subjectively experience something first-hand that is analogous to the patient's emotional experience. This is not just "empathy" in the usual sense, but a deep and physical knowing that may not be identical or analogous in content but equivalent or nearly so in emotional kind. This is the resonance of the analytic relationship. The patient gets the analyst-as-emotional-tuning-fork to "vibrate" to the analyst's equivalent or analogue of the patient's own terrified and/or chaotic frequency. And from the patient's perspective, there is something about knowing that one is so deeply and accurately "known" in a feeling way, that is very powerful and salutary. This is a process of mutual *being* that transcends "being told about" and other forms of verbalization.

What I believe Bion is getting at is that the analyst needs to convey something to the patient *from a deeply personal experience.* This conveyance is not just a "telling about" or a matter of the analyst's disclosure of personal information. It is a physical matter of emotional resonance. One does not—indeed cannot successfully or impactfully—*tell* the patient, but the knowledge that is evoked and lived by the analyst informs the affective quality of the moment as well as the content of what is said in some unconscious fashion. In the language of Bion's (1970) theory, there is *at-one-ment* as one *becomes* the **O** of the patient. "There is an ultimate reality which cannot be known but can only be 'become', that is, it is possible to be at-one with it" (p. 121).

Symington and Symington (1996) convey something of what this feels like or means by putting it in quasi-religious, transcendental language: "the experience of being at one with **O** ... is an experience like incarnation, becoming of the same flesh" (p. 122). They then add: "it is much easier to know about something rather than to become it. Learning about analysis is easy but learning through the living of that aspect of the self, that is, by being it, is not" (p. 123). And, of course, this is as true of the analysts in relation to their own experience, as it is for the analyst in relation to the patient's experience.

I think that what Bion wishes to leave us with is the idea that at the level of the beta screen and the unstructured unconscious, the problem is that of the unbound and uncontained forces that continue to storm through and may disrupt the psyche. From this perspective, effectiveness of our interventions does not come from learning *about* the experience of the other, but perhaps that "learning about" reflects or creates and informs the analyst's own experience, an experience that must be borne and withstood, tolerated, and *become*. And it is this experience of becoming and being that contributes an important component of the therapeutic action in the analysis of non-neurotic patients and states.

While it is traditional to end a deeply conceptual paper such as this with a clinical illustration, readers who have followed my argument will recognize that I am trying to describe something that may be subjectively or intuitively realized, but may defy semantic description. Consequently, I defer to and align myself with Bion (1970), who began his introduction to *Attention and Interpretation* by saying: "I doubt if anyone but a practicing psycho-analyst can understand this book although I have done my best to make it simple" (p. 1).

He goes on to distinguish those who *practice* psychoanalysis and so can rely first hand upon their experience from "those who only read or hear *about* psycho-analysis" (p. 1, original italics) and so must trust the inadequacy and vagaries of "words and verbal formulations designed for a different task" (p. 1). While semantics are perhaps our only or best means of conveyance, they nevertheless are not at all suited to the task at hand. Andre Green (2005) made a similar point when he said that in psychoanalytic writing, good conceptual clinical thinking will allow clinical examples to emerge in the mind of the practicing analyst from the reader's own experience and between the written lines on the page. I hope that what I have written is successful in this regard and has made this chapter useful to readers in similar ways.

I would like to conclude by returning to Bion. Writing in *Cogitations* (1992), he describes a session in which the impact of the patient's discourse is such that he is "forced to have an emotional experience, and … to have it in such a way that [he is] unable to [remember or] learn from it" (p. 220).

Is he describing an experience that felt like an assault on his mind and analytic competence and capacities; an attack on linking? In the next paragraph, he likens it to a similar situation of an incomprehensible outpouring: "out it pours—masses of semi-whispered, disjointed stuff, name after name, some of which I know, some I may be supposed to know, some presumably I cannot be expected to know" (pp. 220–221).

He then asks himself and his readers: "what is it all? Can anyone stem the flood? What interpretation, when there must be so many millions? … Is it the patient proving the superiority of his vision? Is it a modernized discharge? Urination? Flatus? Defecation?" (p. 221).

Seemingly, this, too, might be categorized as an attack on linking, but listen carefully and from another vertex to what Bion then says:

> The essential feeling [*his* feeling] is that nothing can be made of it—there is no selected fact, nothing to make it all cohere. If this is so, then perhaps the essential thing is an emotional situation in which the following features can be distinguished:

1   Feelings of persecution,
2   A mass of apparently unrelated facts,
3   An inability to find a selected fact, or perhaps to believe it would be any good if one could,
4   An inability to see any value in the facts, to regard them as dead particles, bits of faeces.

But surely the point here is a lack of capacity for integrating? Is it that the content is significant? Or is it the cement...? It can be content *and*...

(p. 221)

Significantly, Bion leaves this sentence unfinished; the entry just breaks off. We are left to surmise that the patient has unconsciously evoked in Bion an emotional experience of chaos, of life in a maelstrom without order ("cement"; links) or meaning, all of which is conveyed in the "dot, dot, dot".

It brings to mind the words of Yeats' (1921) poem, *The Second Coming*:

Things fall apart; the centre cannot hold;

Mere anarchy is loosed upon the world

The means of this evocation is the presentation of a de-linked and fragmented discourse. But notice Bion's final question: "Or is it the cement?" Does not his ending, "it can be content *and*...", act upon the reader much as the beta screen does by evocation? For this reader, it leads inexorably to the concluding phrase, "*content and communication*". If the beta screen communicates by evocation of an experience in an object and an object is needed for homeostasis and management of "excess excitation", and words cannot adequately convey that need and the terror and distress that accompanies it, either because the patient is incapable of using words effectively at that moment or language itself is too poor a medium to capture and convey the meaning of what would need to be conveyed, then...

What from one perspective may be seen predominantly as a discharge of excess, unmanageable accretion of stimuli, or an attack on the analyst or the patient's own mind, at the same time from another perspective might be taken in by the analyst as a call for help. As Marshall McLuhan (1964) famously said: "the medium is the message".

Bergstein (2019), commenting on Bion's journal entry, describes Bion as having an emotional experience

[one] that he was unable to [initially] learn from.... Nevertheless, he wonders if one might not, after all, attribute meaning to the similarity between the analyst's predicament and the patient's situation when he is unable to think. In other words, despite the patient's fragmented thinking and the fragmentation that comes along in the analyst's thinking, does

this attack on thinking not tell, in retrospect, some kind of story? The patient's material seems incoherent, but incoherence might be the communication that the patient is trying to convey ... Bion is stressing the operation of the non-psychotic part of the mind in the psychotic patient's personality—that is, the communicative aspect in the part of the personality that seemingly cannot think or communicate.

(p. 101)

Even if the link between patient and analyst is conceptualized as **-K**, where the psychotic part of the personality cannot or does not want to learn from experience and acquire knowledge, there remains within the mind and being of the patient *"the urge to communicate this unwillingness or inability to learn and to know"* (p. 101). That is, there is a non-psychotic part of the patient that is potentially in touch with the chaos and disorder inside and is in search of help in relieving the flood of "stimuli that cannot be mentalized and that remain as an irritating franticness of foreign objects inside his mind and body" (p. 101).

So, even the **-K** link may tell a story:

of a destructive, projective-identification-rejecting relationship between an infant and its primary object (see also Eaton, 2005). This is a relationship where the emotions were too intense for the precarious self and so were experienced as violently attacking it, or else where the self attacked the part of the personality able to perceive the emotions, in order to protect itself from intolerable pain.

(p. 102)

It does not matter whether this problem originated in the self or the object or that certainty about its origin may be and probably is unknowable. What is important is that it is a problem of the link between the two and it is this link that is being unconsciously evoked and recreated in a search for relief.

Bergstein concludes:

this experience in which the patient's and/or analyst's thinking is being attacked in psychoanalysis is thus not only an attack on communication but is also itself a communication. Hence, attacks on linking may be a manifestation of the drive to represent ... or a drive to communicate.

(p. 103)

From the perspective of technique, then, the analyst is always faced with a dual obligation:

- To try to find the potentially communicative meaning and sense of their evoked experience with even the most seemingly destructive, resistant, and oppositional patients,
- To also consider the personal, subjective, potentially conflictual and counter-transferential meaning of that evoked experience.

A patient's attacks on linking, their unique and specific form of "unthinking", may need to be potentially thought about as an unconscious, primal communication meant to convey via evocation a specific mode of being related perhaps to an earlier infantile situation or mode of existence. If the analyst can consider this as a possibility, then the further possibility may exist that the analyst may be able to achieve an analytic vertex from which to consider the situation and ultimately understand or create a plausible, meaningful narrative in relation to the evocation.

Notes

1 I am indebted to Avner Bergstein (2019), who, in his extraordinary book, *Bion and Meltzer's Expeditions into Unmapped Mental Life,* uses this expression to describe a set of feelings unconsciously evoked in him by a patient. An earlier version of this chapter appeared in *Psychoanal. Quart.*, 92: 641–664.
2 There is a sense in which a great deal of Bion's writing, even his early formulations of unconscious group dynamics, attempted to address the problem of how to contain and metabolize the infinitizing, potentially traumatizing, centrifugal forces of raw, being-in-the-world.
3 That is, while the fullness of mental "space" and the phenomena of raw existential Experience are overwhelmingly infinite, that "part" of the psyche that contains the set of representations that we speak of colloquially as our "mind" and its "thoughts" is three-dimensional. Readers may notice – and perhaps will forgive— my use of a spatial metaphor here to try to convey this thought. That I have to resort to something that I know is too concrete, potentially misleading, and literally "false"—the mind is not a "place"—is an example of the limitations of language that I am trying to speak about! For an extended discussion of this problem see Bergstein (2019).
4 I will use the convention of using the capital E to talk about raw existential Experience, which by definition cannot be fully known, but may only "be" or "become" and use the small e to refer to that part of Experience (everyday experience) that can come to be known.
5 Like Freud (see Stanicke et al., 2020), Bion's epistemological reasoning rests within the Western philosophical tradition of thinkers such as Kant and Hume.
6 Laplanche (2002) describes an analogous process when he talks about the unconscious transmission, implantation, and installation of an unknowable sexual desire in the creation of the infant's unconscious.
7 For further discussion, see Levine (2022) and what I have called the Fundamental Epistemological Position.
8 "It is too often forgotten that the gift of speech, so centrally employed, has been elaborated as much for the purpose of concealing thought by dissimulation and lying as for the purpose of elucidating or communicating thought" (Bion, 1970, p. 3).
9 The capacity to accept this trade-off is captured in the concept of primary erotic masochism, a subject discussed at length by Aisenstein (2023).

10 We should also mention Winnicott (1968) here, because the frustration referred to may be that of what he called ego gratification, rather than instinctual gratification or survival need. "Thinking starts as a personal way that the infant has for dealing with the mother's graduated failure of adaptation. Thinking is part of the mechanism by which the infant tolerates both failure of adaptation to ego-need and frustration of instinct producing tension, particularly the former" (p. 213).

11 See also Lombardi (2017).

12 See, for example, Aisenstein (2017): "there are no psychosomatic illnesses: the human being, by definition, is a somatopsychic unity" (p. 76).

13 See also Freud's (1937) paper *On Construction* and Levine (2022) for further discussion.

14 Although the psychotic part of the personality is the designation usually used to indicate the proto-mental or non-neurotico-normal parts of the psyche, I find it an unfortunate choice of words, because it may be taken to imply that we are all in some way "psychotic" or that psychosis is a normal part of infantile development and inheres in all of us throughout our lives. As Green (1986) indicated, we all have our own "private madness", but this is not the same as having a part of our minds that deserves the psychiatric diagnosis of "psychosis".

Following the work of Winnicott (1965) and De Masi (2020), I believe that psychosis is better seen as a particular kind of psychic organization that becomes installed in the mind, turns away from reality, skews psychic functioning toward sensation-generation rather than sense making and is desperately clung to as a last-ditch defense against annihilation anxiety, nameless dread, and the threat of the explosive return of disruptive, traumatizing states of *disintegration*. While psychosis may defend against and embody a great deal of traumatized and traumatizing chaos marked by bizarre objects and failures of representation, I do not believe that psychosis should be viewed as a residue of a normative state of unrepresentation or *unintegration* or assumed to be equivalent to or to denote a mere absence of representations, i.e., the presence of beta elements, drives, not yet transformed sense perceptions, etc. The latter, which may be potential or emergent but not yet formed, are better thought of as making up the majority of the Id, that part of the Id that is not derived from secondary repression of unacceptable, anxiety arousing desires. It is the latter that is normative and universally present and is increasingly being referred to as elements of the *unstructured* or *unrepresented unconscious*.

15 For an extensive discussion of this, see Eshel (2019) and her formulations of "analytic oneness" and "*withnessing*".

16 The attacking, defensive, reality destroying motivations are often implicated in analysts' discussions of Bion's famous 1959 paper and their patients' *Attacks on Linking*.

17 Aisenstein (2017) makes an analogous assertion about somatic discharges: "somatic outcomes are to my mind attempts—presumably last-ditch attempts—to mobilise a reparative aim in 'another', whose value as an object is at the relevant time imperceptible and uncertain" (p. 90).

References

Abel-Hirsch, N. (2019). *Bion. 365 quotes*. Routledge.

Aisenstein, M. (2017). *An analytic journey*. Karnac.

Aisenstein, M. (2023). *Desire, pain and thought*. Routledge.

Bergstein, A. (2019). *Bion and meltzers' expedition into unmapped mental life*. Routledge.

Bion, W.R. (1957). On arrogance. *Int. J. Psychoanal.*, 39, 144–146.

Bion, W.R. (1959). Attacks on linking. *IJPA*, 40, 308–315.

Bion, W.R. (1962). *Learning from experience*. Heinemann.

Bion, W.R. (1965). *Transformations*. Heinemann.

Bion, W.R. (1970). *Attention and interpretation*. Basic Books.

Bion, W.R. (1991). *A memoir of the future*. Karnac.

Bion, W.R. (1992). *Cogitations*. Karnac.

De Masi, F. (2020). *A psychoanalytic approach to treating psychosis*. Routledge.

Eaton, J. (2005). The obstructive object. *Psychoanalytic Review*, 92, 355–372.

Eliot, T.S. (1963). *Collected poems, 1909–1962*. Harcourt, Brace & World.

Eshel, O. (2019). *The emergence of analytic oneness. Into the heart of psychoanalysis*. Routledge.

Freud, S. (1911). Formulations on the two principles of mental functioning. In *S.E.* (Vol. 12, pp. 213–226). Hogarth Press.

Freud, S. (1912). The dynamics of transference. In *S.E.* (Vol. 12, pp. 97–108). Hogarth Press.

Freud, S. (1923/1959). The ego and the id. In *S.E.* (Vol. 19, pp. 1–66). Hogarth Press.

Freud, S. (1937). Constructions in analysis. In *S.E.* (Vol. 23, pp. 255–270). Hogarth Press.

Green, A. (1986). The dead mother. In A. Green (1997), *On private madness* (pp. 142–173). Karnac.

Green, A. (2005). *Psychoanalysis. A paradigm for clinical thinking*, Trans. A. Weller. Free Association.

Junqueira, A., Brito, G., & Levine, H. (Eds.) (2017). *Bion in Brazil*. Karnac.

Laplanche, J. (2002). Starting from the fundamental anthropological situation. In J. Laplanche (2011), *Freud and the sexual* (pp. 99–114). International Psychoanalytic Books.

Levine, H.B. (2022). *Affect, representation and language. Between the silence and the cry*. Routledge/IPA.

Lombardi, R. (2017). *Body-mind dissociation in psychoanalysis. Development after Bion*. Routledge.

McLuhan, M. (1964). *Understanding media. The extensions of man*. McGraw/Hill.

Sandler, J. (1976). Counter-transference and role responsiveness. *Int. Rev. of Psycho-Analysis*, 3, 43–47.

Stanicke, E., Zachrisson, A., & Vetlesen, A.J. (2020). The epistemological stance of psychoanalysis: Revisiting the Kantian legacy. *Psychoanal. Quart.*, 89, 281–304.

Symington, J., & Symington, N. (1996). *The clinical thinking of Wilfred Bion*. Routledge.

Winnicott, D.W. (1960). The theory of the parent-infant relationship. In D.W. Winnicott (1965), *The maturational processes and the facilitating environment* (pp. 37–55). IUP.

Winnicott, D.W. (1965). The psychology of madness. In D.W. Winnicott (1989), *The psychology of madness* (pp. 119–129), Ed. C. Winnicott, R. Shepherd, & M. Davis. Harvard University Press.

Winnicott, D.W. (1968). Thinking and symbol formation. In D.W. Winnicott (1989), *The psychology of madness*, (pp. 213–216), Ed. C. Winnicott, R. Shepherd, & M. Davis. Harvard University Press.

Yeats, W.B. (1921). The second coming. In W.B. Yeats (1956), *The collected poems of W.B. Yeats* (pp. 184–185). MacMillan.

Chapter 4

Bizarre bodily delusions

Béatrice Ithier

Translated by Andrew Weller

This title is inspired by W.R. Bion's notion of the *"bizarre object"* resulting from excessive and specific projective identifications that are characteristic of the hallucinatory functioning of many psychotic personalities. "The patient", Bion writes, "feels he is surrounded by bizarre objects compounded partly of real objects and partly of fragments of the personality" (1958, p. 81). I would like to clarify what might be implied in Freud's suggestion, taken up by Bion, that delusions may be the "equivalents of the constructions which we build up in the course of an analytic treatment, attempts at explanation and cure". Bion agrees, but adds that "some of the patient's delusions were attempts at employing bizarre objects in the service of therapeutic intuition. If so, it may afford a definition of the relationship between delusion and hallucination" (1958, p. 82). I propose to extend this connection by adding trauma and not only environment. Without this dimension, Bion's first approach to psychosis, to which I am referring, although very clear, could remain descriptive and does not go back to its roots. It's a question.

In the approach I am taking, I will start from the idea put forward by Ogden (2021) that "something of the non-self inhabits us". Quoting Freud, he links this non-self to a pressure from biological forces creating "a demand on the mind for work". It seems to me that this non-self could also refer to the pressure exerted by the violence of the trauma in delusions, or even to the pressure of the delusion itself. Both in his early and later work Freud insisted on the kernel of truth in delusions (1907) and on the necessity of construction (1937). I will build on Bion's irrefutable analysis of the "Differentiation of Psychotic and Non-Psychotic Personalities" (1957a), but not without insisting on the infantile aspects that have been assailed by numerous and repeated traumas, sometimes uninterrupted.

Bion, then a Kleinian, started out from "Language and the Schizophrenic" (1953), and in his "Notes on the Theory of Schizophrenia" (1954) elaborated the first foundations of his theory of knowledge, insisting on the particular nature of the psychotic's object-relations marked by splitting, fragmentation of the object and the ego; he conceived only of the negative modalities in psychosis subject to the distortions of evacuative projective identification, as

DOI: 10.4324/9781003534365-4

presented in "On Arrogance" (1957b), and then in "Attacks on Linking" (1959). The discharge of the mind by means of hallucination is accompanied, according to him, by the utilization of the sensory apparatus in the reverse direction. The clinical material of two severely traumatized psychotic patients will attest to the traumatic bodily foundations that validate, as it were, this functioning, resulting in bizarre bodily delusions, the aim of which is also to eject the enacted intrusion of traumatic organs (Luisa) and mechanisms (Marie). It is only with his transcendent conception of the container that Bion advances the notion of primitive catastrophe, when it is absent in the mother. We will see how, in Luisa and Marie, these two approaches to psychosis overlap in the intersubjectivity of the session. This is the aim of this paper.

Orgy of projective identification

Melanie Klein (1946) introduced this fundamental concept in "Notes on Some Schizoid Mechanisms", to designate a particular form of identification establishing the prototype of an aggressive object-relation. It is, in fact, a mechanism inherent to the *paranoid-schizoid position*, by which a projection in phantasy of split-off parts of the subject's personality is carried out into the maternal body, with the aim of controlling the mother from within by arousing, for example, anxieties to do with being shut in and persecuted. At the beginning of his work, Donald Meltzer agreed with this Kleinian conception. But in 1986, in his *Etudes pour une Métapsychologie élargie*, he cites Esther Bick, in highlighting identification processes linked to two-dimensionality (adhesive identification), hence the possible existence of "a psychic structuring prior to the schizo-paranoid position" (p. 243).

I would like to show that it is on the basis of abused bodily zones, or even zones that have actually been intruded upon in reality, that the reversal of projective identification takes place—projection connoting the projection of what the person feels, and has felt, to be bad about themselves, and identification, the identification of these parts or the person with the subject. While Bion, who was still a Kleinian, speaks of instant solutions, promised by the psychotic part to unload the mind of unwanted emotions—something we will see with Luisa and Marie—he describes the psychotic's difficulty in modifying the environment and his haste to evacuate any tension related to the intolerance of frustration. He states that the psychotic resorts to "muscular action … by hallucination, that is by the use of the sensory apparatus in reverse" (1958, p. 83). But why does the psychotic do this? The abundance of the clinical material presented is intended to attest to a conception of the psychotic that places the trauma at the heart of a primitive infantile catastrophe generating psychotic terror.

A few years later, Bion was to propose a mode of functioning based on non-intrusive projective identification, characteristic of the baby who is making his mother experience his psychic states. Thanks to her reverie, the mother will have the task of *"alphabetizing"* the raw elements, sense-impressions—so prominent in psychosis—feelings or impulses that are too painful for the baby, according to his theory of the mind, which differentiates *alpha elements* from *beta elements*. However, the mother of the psychotic closes herself to her child's projections, showing her inability to contain and transform his death anxieties. She may even use her child as a container for her own projective identifications of hatred, in an inverted container/contained functioning. The invalidation of subjective premises by the environment prevents the construction of an acceptable and accepted subjectivity in the incessant internal struggle of the psychotic organization, crystallized around alienating, "obstructive" internal objects (Bion, 1957b, p. 92), constantly accentuated by defensive distortions, and the no less influential dependence on external objects.

In speaking of Luisa and Marie (the former clinging to a bizarre bodily delusion, the latter to numerous delusions, one of which evoked for me a bizarre delusion similar to the one presented in *President Schreiber's Memoirs* [Freud, 1911]), I will highlight the importance of the specific attention given to my emotional experience and feelings, in the juxtaposition, whether split or not, of psychotic and infantile transferences. Their emotional experience and their psychotic effervescence appeared to me to be linked to traumatic situations that were not only uncontained, but reinterpreted in a delusional mode, with the portion of historical truth on which Freud, unlike certain Kleinian authors, insisted. According to him, the delusion reflected "something that has been experienced in infancy and then forgotten returns—something that the child has seen or heard at a time when he could still hardly speak and that now forces its way into consciousness" (Freud, 1937, p. 267). He considered that the analytical task consisted in "liberating the fragment of historical truth from its distortions and its attachments to the actual present day, and in leading it back to the point in the past to which it belongs" (ibid., p. 268).

The recognition of these traumas nourishes the infantile transference and makes the development of the healthy part of the personality possible. In *Psychotic States: A Psychoanalytic Approach*, Herbert Rosenfeld remarked that "in investigating a number of schizophrenic patients it was apparent that psychogenic trauma in infancy played an important role" (1965, p. 166), and in *Impasse and Interpretation* (1987), he cites June Felton's 1985 reference (in a personal communication) to *"osmotic overflow"* or *"pressure"* as an intrauterine physiological process in which the fetus is overwhelmed by feelings or experiences in the mother that she does not want to know about (p. 185). He evokes Bion, according to whom, the mothers of schizophrenics have less tolerance for their infant's projective identifications, feeling persecuted, they decathect the child who will be sensitive to her reaction. In the *Clinical Seminars*, Bion writes:

With this patient it may be very important to show him, when the time comes, that there exists some capacity for affection, sympathy, understanding—not just diagnoses and surgery, not just analytical jargon, but interest in the person. You can't make doctors or analysts—they have to be born.

(1987, p. 18)

The bizarre bodily delusion

I will first talk about Luisa, a woman in her thirties, who took years to come into contact with a trauma consisting of anal violence and terror; this was at the basis of her delusion which she juxtaposed in a very split manner with an intense infantile transference. Luisa was being followed at the same time by a psychiatrist who prescribed medication.

At our first meeting, she described how she walked close to the walls and heard insults all the way to my office, to her psychiatrist's or to the shops because she had to eat, or whenever she made any other necessary outings. She had stopped doing a job where she had felt exposed, and had managed to work from her flat. She told me about what she called her symptom. Her anus wouldn't close, she farted without realizing it, and smelled bad. Her delusion, which had appeared before we met, seemed to have appeared sometime after a hysterectomy, as if the disappearance of her uterus had focused all her attention on the anal area. Her interest, in fact, had been concentrated on her anal sphincter, overdetermining its evacuative function. I had, of course, wondered about this. Even in her bath, bubbles formed from the action of farting, rising to the surface of the water!

Which identificatory projections were thus being rejected through them? What intrusive, devastating, and inverted meaning could be attached to them? Such questions forced themselves on me for a long time. They led me to have to function as a container for her terrifying aspects, which she was expelling. I sought to take them into myself in a less frightening form, giving her the experience of feeling understood and accepted by me, which was a thankless task.

Bion tells us that beta elements arise from an initial sensory impression induced by incoming stimuli, physical in nature, as Grotstein (2007/2016, p. 89) points out, as opposed to alpha elements which are mental. It is as if he then failed to connect the reversed functioning of projective identification to trauma. This is what Bion was to say about this separation:

In saying that, I have made an entirely artificial separation; I have talked about the body and the mind as if they were two entirely different things. I don't believe it. I think that the patient whom you see tomorrow is one, a whole, a complete person. And even if we say, following the rules of grammar that we can observe the body and the mind, in reality such things as a 'body' or a 'mind' do not exist. What exists, is a 'him' or 'her'.

(2005, p. 38)

As she passed by, Luisa said, people took exception to her smell and hurled insults at her, often ending with "It's a disgrace" or "How ugly you are!" She had reconstructed a world full of signs that even included making her pick out the word "fart" in her choice of purchases. She could hear the cries in the street, uttered at any demonstration, as a violent protest against what she called "her bad smell". The extreme conviction of her delusion was impressive. This anus, which she claimed was half-open and unreliable, terrorized her and at the same time she clung to it obstinately.

She accepted the setting of four weekly sessions, and we began her analysis.

She gave me a picture of her father as a violent and paranoid man, with terrifying rages, and of her mother as a depressive, submissive, and unmotherly woman, very involved in a bureaucratic job, and quite absent. Between sessions, she began to write me daily letters that she brought to the session, in which she recorded all her thoughts. She would phone me, beginning "Dear Mother Light". I received hundreds and hundreds of letters during those years. In these often very long letters, she told me about ideas that had come to her after the session, which appeared to me not only as an attempt to extend the relationship with me, as she had done by knitting a scarf for me during a summer holiday, but also to continue the work of thinking in an attempt to reduce the split between her psychotic part and her infantile self.

"Mother Light" was a signifier condensing both the light she seemed to enjoy in the work of thinking in the session, but also a "light" mood in me, which she seemed to be sensitive to, having lived for a long time in the shadow of a terrifying father, and a cold, dead mother, whom she had internalized. We talked about this.

A transport paralysis kept us apart for about a month. When she returned, I suggested that she come five times a week in order to compensate for the missed sessions. She accepted, and this experience constituted a real turning point in our work, underpinning a better continuity. The letters were written to testify to this; they made it possible to approach the traumatic kernel (and kernel of truth) of her delusion.

One day she came up with a dream about a car ride she was taking with her father. The two of them were alone. In the middle of the road, there was a chicken. She had just finished recounting her dream when, without any conscious thought on my part, the words spontaneously came out of my mouth: "You were Daddy's little chicken!" The statement was in the form of an action and afterwards I wondered about it.

We know that Bion considers that the psychotic is in states where they are neither able to sleep nor wake up. The mother or analyst must therefore dream the unthinkable experience of the patient or infant from the experience of her own reverie. This is fundamental. My reverie was enacted. This enacted reverie characterizing Luisa's experience seemed to me to be an unconscious proto-emotional and emotional experience shared in the session and thus reaching its ultimate realization. This is one of the meanings that Bion assigns to O in his later and final thinking.

This also appeared to me to be similar to the emergence of a "chimera", "the chicken", in the sense in which M. de M'Uzan might understand it (2002) and in which I understand it, even if in a very different way. That is to say, a content or an object that emerges from the coalescence of the traces of the two unconsciousness, that of the patient and that of the analyst (Ithier, 2016, 2020). I have often been surprised by these manifestations, which for me resemble enacted reveries, arising from unstoppable dream fragments.

These words triggered a trance in her. She stood up, trembling and shouting at the same time: "This is terrible! terrible!" She wandered around the room in a state of terror, and stopped, contracting herself, screaming and crying, albeit still standing (in the dream, she was sitting). She had just rediscovered the image of a traumatic scene framing the dream, which she began to describe to me.

Faced with her agitation and terror, I inevitably wondered about the impact of the violence that my intervention had provoked. It was undeniable that Luisa had been "*found*" here in the ambivalent sense given to it by Winnicott (1969), but *too* found (while, on the other hand, the despair of not being found can arise). This questioning of myself was in response to my unfiltered approach to the kernel of a self that had never ceased to be hidden and protected.

The scene:

When she was about two and a half years old, she was in the car behind the wheel, "driving" with her father behind her; she was pressed up against him. She felt something hard behind her. Her father was excited and had an erection. He drove her into a clearing, undressing her hurriedly, partially succeeding in an attempt at sodomy. Some walkers surprised them and shouted: "This is a shame, you don't do that with a child, we will report it". This could throw light on the shame and clamor of voices she heard whenever she left her house, or even inside her flat when she felt sexually aroused and, in identification with the aggressor, masturbated anally, and in other ways. She remembered that when she came home in her stained and soiled dress, her mother, seeing her in this mess and all dirty, had become angry and called her "ugly", which she kept hearing in the voices of her delusion. This memory stunned her. However, the delusion, or rather its shreds, had not yet given way to the obstinacy of the splitting. It was only gradually, when she returned home and heard the voice of a loving mother speaking tenderly to her child on the other side of the bedroom wall, that she was able to project her infantile self into the child by projecting me into this mother, thus giving a very concrete, sensory content to the infantile transference that she had experienced with me. It was as if psychic reality had to be embodied in concrete reality in order to be introjected.

This subjection to the concrete, so prevalent in the psychotic psyche, invaded by saturating beta elements, which Bion characterizes as an "inability to dream", can foment the chimera in the process of depersonalization depicted by the analyst's reverie, especially as the state of unison here is underpinned by traumatic meshes (Ithier, 2020).

Marie's skin

I want to turn now to Marie, in her thirties, and to explore some aspects of her delusions, delusions that have disappeared without medication. From the beginning, I was overcome by an experience of "at-one-ment" or "unison" (Bion, 1970) that I felt in the dynamics of our incredibly intense emotional exchanges, and in a state of union or communion. I had never seen anyone cry like that. I was both overwhelmed and permeated by it.

I am going to explore the varied spectrum of her psychotic states associated with a raw infantile transference by revisiting, in the here-and-now, the trajectory and intensity of the identificatory, differentiated, and even trans-psychic projections (Grotstein, 2007/2016) that occupied, in the interpsychic communication, such a prominent place. The diversity of states and parts, and the intensity of the register of projective identification, seemed to me to define the valency of the exchanges with her. Because of the emotional expressiveness of her affects, the variety of her splitting, and the importance of her defenses, particularly manic defenses, this work was part of a complex and contrasted alchemy that she sometimes referred to as a "journey of the soul". After four years of Lacanian analysis, she had consulted a magnetizer in the provinces and an exorcist of the archbishop.

During our *first meeting*, I was immediately struck by the discrepancy between the apparent charm of her face and the emotional violence that inhabited it. As we greeted each other, I could already sense her powerful sense of distrust.

Once she had entered my office, she looked at me very deeply and inspected everything around her with great insistence. Even before we had sat down, she said to me: "When you opened the door, I thought you looked like my analyst, fragile like her. She was blonde like you". She stared at me and continued: "While I was waiting next door, I found you had some beautiful objects. There were a lot of things. It's substantial".

I could hear her greedy demand and, in the background, her anxiety about emptiness.

No sooner had we sat down than her face turned red and suddenly looked like a mask or an expressionist painting. The atmosphere in my office was then one of great tension and terror. "It's awful", she said. She was struggling hard not to cry. Her face turned very red. "I feel empty. I've managed to create a character for myself, that's all". She added, "The job I'm doing is terrible. There are acts of vandalism and malice". She had found blood-stained sanitary towels on her chair, dead mice in her drawers, the metal legs of her table sawed off. She had also found rubbish on her floor of the building where she lived. I could hear the delusion.

She continued: "I was in analysis, I couldn't get out of it".

I thought about the probable violence of her unreceived projective identifications. *She continued: "I am afraid of emotional failure".* I found this formulation striking.

"I have had to struggle with this. I am afraid that my soul is going to go to hell. I would like an analyst, but someone I can trust."

I clearly heard an analyst, and I understood that she was showing me both that she was still expecting an emotional success from the experience of analysis, but above all that she had struggled a lot, including with delusions, against these failures, no longer trusting her analyst, as in her emotional environment in childhood. I said to her: "Yes, someone with whom you can hope that there will be no emotional failure, so that you can get out of this repetition that gives you this feeling of emptiness and damnation".

I thought about the exorcist of the archbishop!

This intervention seemed to me a little flat, whereas I wanted it to be synthetic; I should have linked the emotional failure more with the feeling of damnation by showing her that, despite the new failure with her analyst, she was still expecting an emotional experience from the analysis. I recalled the shock that the violence of her suffering, depicted on her face and embodied in her voice, had aroused in me at the outset, and which was interfering with my thought processes by slowing them down. I also felt a massive identificatory projection in me.

She continued: *"My father was never around and I was afraid of him. My mother was not affectionate at all.* I'm like an autistic spot, like someone in a concentration camp". She remained silent.

"Autistic spot", the formulation was striking, and I said to her:

> It's as if you were telling me that nothing had ever opened up for you in your parents' feelings, and that everything had remained on the surface in the analysis, without you feeling alive in your analyst's mind? Now you feel shut in, suffering with these fears and all these unacknowledged emotional needs.

I linked this up in myself with the feeling of having intervened in a flat way, while feeling compelled to intervene in a richer way, as if I myself were shut in.

I was drawing on what she was already making me feel strongly. She replied: "I was feeling bad and she didn't say anything, just: 'I'll be waiting for you then', for the next session. I gave her my money, like to the taxman". She continued:

> Apart from my parents, there is a man I am deprived of. He doesn't respond to my requests. I continue to fantasize. I have always lived like a dream. What scares me is my destiny. I am afraid of everyone. I am also afraid that I will murder you.

It was as if she was beginning to understand a bit how she functioned because there was someone listening to her. This fear of murdering me reminded me of Bion's analysis of aggression in psychosis which, according to him, is but "the outward expression of an explosive projective identification", by virtue of which the patient's murderous hatred, together with the "bits" of his personality, is scattered far and wide into the real objects surrounding him (1958, p. 84), namely bizarre objects comprising hatred and murderous consciousness.

I saw her, violently red, the skin of her face becoming more and more like the rough thickness of a mask, like the skin of a character in an expressionist painting and, more realistically, testifying to the violence of parental projective trans-identifications. I felt she was powerfully inhabited by mixed and paroxysmal feelings. Her fear of murdering me made me experience the murderous relationship with the mother, on the model of her mother with her. I told her that for the moment, she did not trust me enough to be able to change this repetition, especially as I was also a woman, but I felt myself inhabited by a great deal of gentleness and I asked her: "Would it be true to say that you experience me as a threat to your emotional needs?" She replied:

> It's traced out. I'm afraid I can't defend myself; my head line is broken and my luck line is non-existent. I've rushed into the analysis. What I know, I know in spite of myself. I know very little. I have nothing.

"*Rushed in*", indeed, because of tropisms and identificatory projections. I also thought that with her "*broken head line*" she was bringing me her madness. She seemed to be explaining to me that she felt deprived, which she also seemed to imagine as an intellectual exercise of which she said she was incapable. And I had the impression that she was telling me more than anything else how she felt locked up and unable to think. I told her this. She remained motionless and added: "I have deprived myself of every little cake for this analysis. I prayed. I prayed a lot to the Blessed Virgin. I understand very little".

The idea came to me that she was asking me to help her think (and rather quickly), and I said to her: "It is as if, in this analysis, there had been too much effort to understand and not enough experiences of feeling heard, so in looking for the Blessed Virgin you were looking for an omnipotent mother to support you". And I added: "Perhaps you also have difficulty understanding me?" I began to think that if she opened herself up to me, she would also be opening herself to immeasurable suffering within her.

Once again, I could see her (her face was crimson), making a very big effort not to cry, and then she rested her bust on a round pedestal table, near where she was sitting, and wrapped her arms around it. Suddenly I could see the deficient container. She cried, hiccupping, overcome by an enormous amount of child's sorrow, a baby's sorrow. I felt and understood that she was showing me—with her face hidden and her arms wrapped around the pedestal table—how much she had had to contain and support herself with these anxieties and this considerable depression. She cried for a long time. Then I told her that she was showing me that it was very important for her to feel accepted by sharing her pain and grief, which she had kept inside her for so long.

After a while, she sat up. She began to inspect things around her again. With the new look on her face, I felt as if I was in front of a new expressionist canvas. Her gaze swept over every wall of my office. While she was facing me, she turned around, inspecting the bookcase behind her for a long time, without paying attention to me anymore. She had entered me and was examining my interior with incredible insistence.

At the level of feelings, it was something quite extraordinary, but I linked it to the closedness of the parents and particularly of the mother, of which I took the full measure, and during this reverie, like a rapid dream fragment, I thought of my mother's closedness, and then I heard her say: "Ovid, Metamorphoses".

This book had caught her eye. I heard this title as a very concrete communication, as a request for transformation, for metamorphosis rather, I wasn't forgetting the Holy Virgin! O void, metamorphosis. I thought: "Metamorphose this void".

I told her that she was wondering if I had the capacity to transform this emptiness in her.

She stared at me intently. This is what she would do at the beginning of the sessions for a long time. I took notes while watching her. *She told me a little later that seeing my hand on the paper helped her to follow her train of thought*; I told myself that it also helped mine!

She left.

Due to the intensity of this first meeting, her call half an hour later did not surprise me. She wanted to work with me. I had seen her arrive with this red expressionist-style face, composed of a superposition of layers, corresponding to layers of psychic states turning into masks. It was very spectacular. Sometimes her face was full of anguish, sometimes she was struggling hard not to cry. It was as if she was exaggeratingly, even desperately, containing this emotional violence within her. From that first interview, I felt that I was the repository of certain anxieties, the texture of which seemed to me to be very traumatic. Her grief reflected her suffering from having had to experience them, while feeling locked up and intoxicated by them. It was as if she had brought me a state of anguish and suffering at its peak.

This is how Marie came into my life as an analyst. Salomon Resnik (personal communication) considered that psychotics end up, to a certain extent, being part of the analyst's family, his/her internal family, certainly!

During the **second interview**, she was quick to express her fear that I would do *"bad things"* to her and that she *"wouldn't be able to defend herself"*.

I reminded her of the fear she had of murdering me and the link that might exist with this fear. She also told me about *her feeling of "being very low", of not existing for me because her social level was lower than mine.*

This communication made me think of the silence and impassivity of her analyst, which she no doubt experienced as a form of contempt for her psychic life, repeating the distance of her mother, and the absence of her father. But in the *"here-and-now"* she was also expressing to me her suffering at feeling that her way of thinking was inferior to mine.

It was only in the **third interview** that she was able to tell me, as she began, that she *"was feeling a bit more herself"*, but that she was so vulnerable, like *"a homeless wandering child"*.

Thus, an authentic infantile transference was expressed. She added: *"Coming here opens the door for me a lot, my mind is more available to hear a little bit of something. What I have experienced is abominable"*.

She *"was feeling a little bit more herself"*, she told me, which I understood to mean the relief experienced by the interpretation of the projective identification that restored her identity, and allowed a child in distress to express herself. As for the "abominable" nature of what she had experienced, I had no doubt about it, given the traumas, their invalidation by the environment, and their identificatory consequences weaving their way through psychotic pathology. I thought it was time for this wandering child to start an analysis with me. I offered her a reduced fee for four sessions a week, saying that I would increase it when her situation improved. She accepted this with a mixture of surprise and relief. I felt I had to be receptive to both the infantile transference, as she was beginning *"to hear a little something"*, and the psychotic transference. I thought that this proposal for a reduced price might lead to some difficulties; for example, she might have the fantasy that I was accusing her of stealing from me, but her suffering deserved an adjusted treatment setting. It was a vector of renewal and transformation.

In the **first session**, she told me about all the *"terrible irritations"* she had had in her body *since she was a child, sore throats, ear aches, ear infections, etc.*

While she was telling me about them, I had the feeling that she was a very sick and small child who was asking me for help, and to whom I had to open my arms psychically. She also told me about the *eczema that had turned her into what she called a "blood ball"*. She was scarlet-faced and upset when she told me about it. We were immersed in a past that was indistinguishable from the present. I really felt that I had to look after this child intensely.

"I had my scalp shaved; the doctors couldn't treat me. They put cardboard sleeves on my arms", she told me. When she spoke about her arms, I thought again about this child to whom I had to open my arms psychically. I was impressed by what she was able to elicit in me on a massive scale. In the same session, she spoke about her former job, which had a certain creative quality and which she had had to give up because she was so overwhelmed by her anxieties and her problematic relationship with reality: "I could never achieve my dreams, I started from scratch, and I started from almost nothing".

I told her, making a link with the analysis that we were starting, that "it was perhaps the same impression she had of feeling helpless on starting this analysis with me", and then I added that she had been able to succeed in this profession; even if it had been too difficult for her to continue on her own, now there were two of us to move forward together. I felt like I was taking a child by the hand.

At the ***next session*** *she told me about her "most terrible anxieties" and mentioned this bizarre delusion. "There's a great racket going on in my house. I hear noises in my corridor at night. In the back bedroom, my feet are grabbed by the wall and then it falls sharply on the bed. There are vibrations and I emit terrible screams. I am very afraid of being buried alive. I can't blame my parents".*

Her delusion reminded me of one of Schreiber's delusions. He was attached during his infancy and childhood to all sorts of blunt and sadistic devices, invented by his father's perverse madness, and was unable to subjectivize the damage caused by the object, due to its idealization. The delusion transformed him into a pleasure-seeking and persecuting God. This was not far from the alternating phases of sadistic restraint and seductive gratification that marked his education. Here, it was the cardboard sleeves and straps with which she was attached to her cot to prevent her from scratching herself that played the role of Schreiber's father's restraining devices, with the same idealizing prohibition concerning the parents.

In that same session, she told me for the first time that "she felt very bad about leaving me".

I thought then: with the idea of being alone with this madness inside her. All this excitement also without a container, without a "psychic skin" (Anzieu, 1985).

I told her *that she was afraid of being faced with all these anxieties when she left me.*

At the ***third session***, *when there was a crushed cat in a pool of blood in front of the door of my building, she projected herself into this cat which seemed to represent her moribund infantile self and, when she arrived, expressed to me her panic that I would kill her, because I would have had enough of her and because I would find her too slow.*

Because of her paranoid anxieties, which Waelder (1951) described as anxieties related to what is "denied", I chose not to refer her to a psychiatric colleague for medication. I felt that she might be too afraid that she would be considered crazy or be made even crazier, that she would be robbed of her sense of identity, or that she might think that I wanted to poison her via someone else. She had a lot of bronchitis and moreover treated herself exclusively with oligo- elements and clay, which she put in her mouth and in her anus at night, so that she would be well stopped up, as her father had asked her to do: *"Above all", he said, "keep things to yourself, don't tell us anything about your problems. Your mother won't stand for it, your mother can't hear that".*

I felt confronted by her terror having to do with expressing to me her anxieties that clung to her throat, tongue, and lips, as she said in the very first sessions. She was so afraid of making me anxious or crazy by communicating them to me, or that to defend myself from her, I would have her locked up. At the same time, she had the capacity to express to me with great spontaneity her needs as a baby and as a little girl. Very split contents were expressed in parallel. When she realized what she had projected into me, she was terrified about having made me carry the weight of her anxieties. She immediately tried to repair me. I understood that this was a very complicated situation for her.

Her father used to say to her: "We can't stand your problems".

In fact, she felt the opposite. She couldn't stand her parents' problems. It was obvious to me that this was what she was "showing" with her mask-face. It was their own problems that she was reflecting back to them and that they could not bear.

The extraordinary power of her infantile transference seemed to me to be the best source of help. To begin this work with a certain feeling of security, I took support from an early communication she had made to me about one of the innumerable employees who had taken care of her, some of whom I later knew to be abusive: "With Josephine, it wasn't terrible (as with the others), she gave us food". So, I thought, if she felt I was here, present, feeding her with understanding and meaning, her psychotic anxieties would gradually subside.

Her mother appeared to me to be undemanding of the people she entrusted Marie to. During her absence, her father, who had returned unexpectedly, had found Marie, a baby, tied up in the cradle, screaming and deprived of food. It was precisely in this state that she had presented herself to me in the first interviews and sessions, emotionally and psychologically speaking.

I understood the deep reason for the "intolerable suffering" (as she called it) that she had experienced during her first professional job, in which she found herself, in effect, trapped in positions from the past. Deprived of the contact of her mute analyst, who did not offer any thinking to her, she had had to relive her torturous experience in her cradle, whereas her professional activity seemed to have corresponded previously to a certain capacity to review the objects to which her gaze had clung, as a baby, in order to escape from the emptiness and the distress.

I took into account the insistence of Marie's father that she should "force herself to keep everything to herself, because her mother wouldn't stand for it" and considered that it was necessary to bear the inevitable and necessary violence of her projections in the field of the sessions. On several occasions I was confronted with her cries, even her screams, which again reminded me of Schreiber's screams when he was with Flechsig. They occurred after crying, first acutely and then in an irrepressible climax, bringing out the violence of the excitement and then of the suffering. I once feared that a gas employee who had come to read the meter would call the police on hearing such screams. I thought it was important for them to be expressed, accepting them, even at their most acute point. And if I sometimes suffered from it, it seemed fundamental to me to receive the climax of this suffering, because once accepted and then shared, it became bearable and was gradually transformed.

Faced with her propensity for massive projective identifications, it seemed to me that I had to deal with the psychotic parts associated with the severe traumas of her childhood or early childhood that had generated terrors reflecting the fact that she had never had someone to reassure her, someone who was there and to whom she could communicate these experiences. Like Klein, Bion considers that the whole future development of the personality will depend on the existence of an object, the breast. If it does not exist, the result is a disaster which, in the end, takes the form of a loss of contact with reality, apathy or mania. Its essential quality is aggressiveness and hatred.

Conclusion

In this paper I wanted to describe and illustrate a receptive and emotionally rich approach to psychosis by unfolding the different accents of these bizarre bodily delusions, driven by the overflow of projective identifications fomenting these bizarre objects populating the psychotic world. The infantile transference, punctuated by powerful affects projected into the analyst, intersects with the projective identifications arising from the psychotic organization. The analyst must understand, as did Bion, that *meanings are double meanings*; for the psychotic, it is a matter, in my opinion, of restoring the meaning of what he or she has experienced and of which the two protagonists in the field have become the guarantors. This question of sharing and recognition seems fundamental to me.

Two approaches to psychosis overlap in Bion. One is Kleinian, leading him to conclude his approach to the "Development of Schizophrenic Thought" (1956) with these words: "experience ... has convinced me that the treatment of psychotic personality will not be successful until the patient's destructive attacks on his ego, and his substitution of projective identification for repression and introjection, have been worked through" (p. 42). The other, from a

later period, is part of the alpha/beta model, where the beta elements correspond to a kind of sensitive, emotional impression of O, or, as Grotstein
describes it: "represent the initial sensory impression of the intersection of O
with our emotional receptors—our emotional sentinels on the lookout" (2007/
2016, pp. 87–88).

According to Bion, the maternal function as a negative container can, in
psychosis, refuse to receive and alphabetize beta elements. In this case, an
internalization of this object transforms it into an "obstructive" object, linked
to the primitive catastrophe. Could they then be degraded alpha elements
rather than beta elements? Or could they still be the balfa elements mentioned
by Ferro (2017). Or even these strange objects, coming from a beta screen, or
rather from an alpha screen, which are also degraded, leading the subject to
project while expecting the contents to be rejected, an attitude so obvious in
Luisa and Marie, and other similar patients? While Bion considered beta
elements as sensory impressions resulting from the impact of incoming physical and non-mental stimuli, Luisa and Marie both bring us the distortions
of the bodily underpinning of the psyche, linked to traumatic intrusions per-
petrated by the environment and delusional factors, giving rise to the dom-
ination of inverted projective identifications.

I have tried to demonstrate the evacuative projective use of proto-emotions
and emotions, as well as of the mind, in psychosis. These result from hate-
filled maternal projective identifications, in connection with the anti-emo-
tional and anti-depressive use of the psychotic organization because of identification with the internal figures that are most hostile to emotions and
feelings, for fear of the repetition of traumas and anxieties of breakdown. In
this struggle, the infantile transference which is frequently fought against
because of the unbearable nature of separations, constitutes the best ally in
the progressive neutralization of the psychotic aspects. This is how Marie
spoke to me one day, saying: "You know, where once there were souls who
used to take my legs in the walls at night, I am now sitting on your lap and
saying: 'my mother'". We can think here of what Bion tells us of the pre-
conception having found a realization of a present breast in waiting: "in the
walls at night, I am now sitting on your lap and saying my mother".

To conclude, I have tried to discuss in Bion's first theory the recourse
through muscular movements to evacuative projective identification, which is
silent with respect to the intrusive traumatic dimension suffered. On the other
hand, Bion conceives beta elements as sensory impressions resulting from
physical and not mental stimuli. The recognition of trauma is very present in
his second theory with the notions of terror and primitive catastrophe in
psychosis, but also with the notions of "at-one-ment", the emotional sharing
to the point of being in "unison", which leads the analyst to become the
emotional reality of the analysand (Bion, 1970). This constitutes one of the
meanings of O, allowing access to the deepest affects (Ithier, 2020), which
alone are capable of transforming the psychotic construction. The experience

with Luisa and Marie showed me the necessity of an emotional and affective survey of these territories, allowing for the transformation of their narcissistic tragedies in an intersubjective weaving whose "at-one-ment" or the fact of being one, leads to the ultimate reality (O) (Bion, 1965).

References

Anzieu, D. (1985/1989). *The skin ego.* Yale University Press.

Bion, W.-R. (1953). Language and the schizophrenic. In P. Heimann, M. Klein., & R. Money-Kyrle (Eds.) (1985), *New directions in psychanalysis.* Routledge.

Bion, W.-R. (1954). Notes on the theory of schizophrenia. In *Second thoughts* (1967, pp. 23–35). Heimann.

Bion, W.R. (1956). Development of schizophrenic thought. In *Second thoughts* (1967, pp. 36–42). Heimann.

Bion, W.R. (1957a). The differentiation of the psychotic from the non-psychotic personalities. *International Journal of Psychoanalysis*, 38(3–4), 266–275.

Bion, W.R. (1957b). On arrogance. *International Journal of Psychoanalysis*, 39, 144–146.

Bion, W.R. (1958). On hallucination. *International Journal of Psychoanalysis*, 39(5), 81.

Bion, W.R. (1959). Attacks on linking. In *Second thoughts* (1967, pp. 93–109). Heimann.

Bion, W.R. (1965). *Transformations: Change for learning to growth.* Tavistock.

Bion, W.R. (1970). *Attention and interpretation.* Tavistock.

Bion, W.R. (1987). *Clinical seminars and other works.* Karnac.

Bion, W.R. (2005). *The Italian seminars.* Routledge.

de M'Uzan, M. (2002). *La chimère des inconscients.* Presses Universitaires de France.

Ferro, A. (2017/2020). *Pensées d'un psychanalyste irrévérencieux.* Ithaque.

Freud, S. (1907). Delusions and dreams in Jensen's 'Gradiva'. In *S.E.* (Vol. 9, pp. 1–95). Hogarth.

Freud, S., (1911). Psychoanalytic notes on an autobiographical account of a case of paranoia. In *S.E.* (Vol. 12, pp. 9–82). Hogarth.

Freud, S. (1937). Constructions in analysis. In *S.E.* (Vol. 23, pp. 255–269). Hogarth.

Grotstein, J. (2007/2016). *Un rayon d'intense obscurité.* Ithaque.

Ithier, B. (2016). The arms of the chimeras. *International Journal of Psychoanalysis*, 97 (2).

Ithier, B. (2020). Boundaries and depths of the oneiric. *International Journal of Psychoanalysis*, 101(5).

Klein, M. (1946). Notes on some schizoid mechanisms. *International Journal of Psychoanalysis*, 27, 99–110.

Meltzer, D. (1986). *Studies in extended metapsychology: Clinical applications of Bion's ideas.* Clunie Press. [*Etudes pour Une Métapsychologie Elargie: Applications Cliniues des Idées de Wilfred R. Bion* (2006). Editions du Hublot, Larmor-Plage.]

Ogden, T. (2021). *Coming to life in the consulting room: Toward a new psychoanalytic sensibility.* Routledge.

Rosenfeld, H. (1965). *Psychotic states: A psychoanalytic approach.* Maresfield.

Rosenfeld, H. (1987). *Impasse et interpretation.* Routledge.

Waelder, R. (1951). The structure of paranoïd ideas: A critical survey of various theories. *International Journal of Psychoanalysis, 32*, 167–177.

Winnicott, W.D. (1969/1958). *Through paediatrics to psychoanalysis. Collected papers.* Tavistock.

Chapter 5

Reaching the body through the mind

A model and its implications

Rudi Vermote

Introduction: The infinite distance between psychoanalysis and the mysterious body

It is not difficult to find some figures on the internet that give one a feel of the infinity of the human body. Our bodies are a part of the stream of life on earth. Our body consists of some 60 trillion cells and 10 million ATP molecules per second per cell are needed as our energy supply, as in all living beings. The cells of all living beings replicate by DNA. This is strikingly similar—the DNA in flies for instance is actually 95% the same as that found in humans. All cells communicate within the body and with the environment. We could paraphrase Winnicott in saying that there is no such thing as a body, only a body/environment unit. This communication happens at many levels: electromagnetic, biomagnetic, hormonal, neurohormonal, feelings, non-verbal expressions, smells, warmth. This enormous communication happens even before any language is present. When we take only the neuro-chemical connections, we know that there are some hundred trillion existing neuronal connections in the human brain. This is at least 1000 times more than the number of stars in our galaxy. The number of possible neuronal connections is infinite. Activity in the body can be measured by looking at the blood flow, a human body having 97,000 km of blood vessels. Our microbiome has 39 trillion cells. It is a body that we carry with us and we cannot live without it. Imagine the highly complex task of the immune system to see which microorganisms should be attacked and where. Luckily, the mind does not have to control all these things. Actually, the fragile mind does not give us an accurate reflection of the world—it creates an illusory three-dimensional model of the infinite world. For instance, the mind does not perceive that everything is emptiness and energy and it has no feeling that the earth turns around the sun at 107,000 km per hour, the sun itself moving within this galaxy at 720,000 km per hour, while the galaxy moves at 201 million km/h.

Against these few data, we may wonder whether it is possible to talk about the infinite body with some poor concepts of psychoanalysis that are still at a

DOI: 10.4324/9781003534365-5

sensuous and descriptive level—not even predictive or abstract or computational.

Talking about the body

This verbal descriptive approach is problematic in another way as well. Verbal thinking creates a dichotomy between "body" and "mind". The real body is however a kind of "brain-heart-skin-gut...-body" (BHSGIbody). Mind is just one frail function of the BHSGIbody. This organization of networks shows that the mind is not only in the brain but all over the BHSGIbody. Verbal thinking is not fit for apprehending the BHSGIbody. We are confronted with a "wall of language". This verbal thinking about the BHSGIbody shows us the limits of the mind. Verbal thought does not reach this body, it may well be possible that we will have to de-structure language to make a contact with the BHSGIbody possible. The body (soma) that our verbal thinking mind creates is a construction/projection of the mind, this is in contrast to the real BHSGIbody—das Leib which has an existence independent of the mind's construction/projection.

Some basic psychoanalytic models of the mind and its relationship with the body

Psychoanalytic models stress the unconscious side of the mind or psychic functioning.

In his topical model, Freud (1915) described the characteristics of the functioning of the dynamic unconscious, based on displacement and condensation. In his structural model, he mentions several kinds of this unconscious functioning: the unconscious ego, the repressed unconscious, the unrepresentable unconscious barred by primal repression. In his "New Introductory Lectures", Freud (1933) changed the egg drawing of his structural model—it is no longer closed, but the bottom consisting of the basic unrepresentable unconscious is figured as open to the body.

Klein (1935, 1946) extended the unconscious mind beyond the visual boundaries of a person by her notion of projective identification, where in phantasy parts of one's own mind are put into others and are controlled there. She saw the mind as a permanent stream of unconscious phantasies that integrate perceptions, memories, and the way we deal with the world. By their origin, most of these phantasies are embodied.

From his work with psychotics, Bion (1962) knew that such unconscious phantasy functioning is not evident. In his theory of thinking, he described beta-elements which are not yet mental and are unknown and unknowable. Somatic sensations and perceptions exist at this beta level before they enter the mind and become alpha elements. This alpha functioning needs to be ignited by a caregiver who transforms the beta-elements by reverie, so that they may become thoughts/emotions of different degrees of abstraction. When the baby/patient takes these in, his own alpha-function can get started.

In contrast to Freud, Bion (1961) started however from an open, undifferentiated, and psychophysical protomental matrix, a field concept to which he would return later in developing his concept of O. Nevertheless, during his elaboration of the model of the mind described above, he saw the mind as existing within a person, not unlike Freud and Klein.

Winnicott (1949) took a different point of view and did not see the mind as something internal—but from the start as in-between. In his idea, the mind only exists in relation with other minds or persons. Moreover, the mind in Winnicott is not distinct from the psyche-soma and only exists in itself as a defense against a trauma and then becomes a mind-psyche instead of a mind-psyche-soma. Then the mind-psyche closes and exists outside of the relationship.

These are just a few of the many psychoanalytic models of the mind, that all have a specific idea about the body-mind link at their base.

An integrative model

For clinical use, it is possible to schematize what has been said so far by a zonal model of psychic functioning based on Bion's model of the mind (Vermote, 2013, 2014, 2019a, b, 2020). This model makes it possible to integrate several psychoanalytic, neuroscientific, and philosophical approaches. Over the years it has been applied to psychopathology, psychoanalytic technique, art, love, philosophy, but it would lead us too far to elaborate this here.

The model is based on an application of Matte Blanco's (1988) concept of the infinite/finite to Bion's model of psychic functioning. Employing this model we may discern three zones or levels: Reasoning, Transformation in K, and Transformation in O.

The first zone is the zone of Reason. This is the zone of finite, conscious verbal thought—perfect for operational problem solving. It accounts for 5% of our psychic functioning and is especially good for practical problems with few variables. For relational, emotional, and spiritual matters however, this approach is less efficient, though it is idealized in our society. Reason is not of much use during psychoanalytic sessions because it blocks free association and free-floating attention, and because it precludes contact from the third zone.

The second zone is the zone of Transformation in Knowledge. Transformation in knowledge is a mixed finite/infinite functioning that is largely unconscious. Freud discovered its characteristics in studying dreams. It is automatic, effortless and goes on day and night. Bion called it reverie and waking dream thought. It also corresponds to Kleinian phantasy and is not unlike Freud's (unconscious) ego-functioning. It may be linked neuroscientifically with the Default Mode Network (DMN) (Mason et al., 2007; Carhart-Harris & Friston, 2010). Symbolizing, mentalizing, phantasy, creativity, dreaming and dream thoughts, and representations all originate in this zone of effortless psychic functioning. This zone is by nature self-centered and is the origin of anxiety. Over the last two decades, most psychopathology has been explained and dealt with in terms of the functioning/dysfunction of T (K). When something does not get symbolized or mentalized it is seen as pathogenic. This is still the main explanation of, and psychoanalytic approach to, psychosis, trauma, psychosomatics, and anorexia nervosa.

The third zone is the zone of O and transformation in O. This zone is outside verbal thought and representations and hence infinite and undifferentiated. It is a zone without distinctions between internal/external, self/other, and body/mind. Nevertheless, we can conceive some a-sensuous empty patterns in this zone, or to use an expression of Augustine: forms in potentio. They are not yet expressed in sensuous forms and are therefore mute, in the dark so to speak. At the deep, fully infinite level is a silent "Dasein", a wordless pure experience—where direct intuitive contact is possible.

The relationship between the three zones of psychic functioning

The first zone is in competition with the second zone: it is not possible to think logically and freely associate at the same time. The contact with the third zone is barred by verbal thinking of which the first zone consists and which is in different degrees also present in the second zone. It is not possible to go by reasoning (first zone) and even by reverie (second zone) to the third zone. The movement is always from O to K, from the third to the second zone and to the first zone. This may happen when these zones are in a receiving mode, but not by deliberately searching for contact. The contact of the third zone with the second zone cannot be wanted, but it may be facilitated by decreasing the functioning of the second zone. The third zone shows no distinction external/internal, mind/body, self/other, but we cannot apprehend it. It is pure experience, intuition (knowing without knowing, direct contact). Although we cannot reach the third zone by an activity of the second zone, the second zone may "catch" what comes from the third zone by its spontaneous mental processing or T(K) and put it into forms, which may be visual or may employ one of the other senses. This movement from the third to the second zone can be facilitated, by being as close as possible to the third zone, to the infinite. Techniques such as "no memory, no desire, no understanding, no senses" (Bion, 1970) facilitate this transition by giving no "food" to the second zone. In this way the functioning of the second zone decreases and also gets more open. Second zone functioning always goes on, day and night (waking dream thought)—but when more open to the third zone, the second zone is functioning more freely and is less self-centered. It may also be possible that elements from the third zone reach the first zone, bypassing the second zone. This may result in a kind of pure experience or pure consciousness.

The body-mind relationship seen from this zonal metapsychology

The body-mind relationship can be looked at from the zonal model. In the first finite zone of psychic functioning, the rational verbal thinking mode represents the body and creates a difference between mind and body by these representations.

In the second zone of the model, we may discern several degrees of the mixture infinite/finite or differentiatedness/undifferentiatedness. In the upper layer of the second zone, where there is still more finite functioning—the difference between the mind and body is less sharp than in the first pure finite zone but representations are more embodied living phantasies than in the first zone. In a so-called middle layer of the second zone, with more infinite than finite functioning (relatively speaking) the body-mind difference is disappearing. This is, for instance, present in the background-primal mother experience (Vermote, 2019c); it is a mental-physical experience which is not well differentiated. In an even "deeper" layer of the second zone, closer to infinite functioning, the differences totally disappear. It is a state which is called in the Eastern philosophies of mind: no-mind, no body. The third infinite zone is a zone that we cannot talk about or represent. It is totally outside of, and beyond, verbal thought and is a direct experience which is in the "bodymind"—but words make no sense at this level of experience. It is a body mind unity, but in a state which is outside of discriminative verbal thoughts and words.

Bion's psychosomatic and somatopsychic functioning

In medicine a difference is usually made between psychosomatic and somatopsychic effects and diseases. Psychosomatic diseases for instance, are diseases in which psychic stress plays a large role. In these diseases psychic stress can affect the skin, heart, immune, or gastro-intestinal systems. By contrast, somatopsychic diseases are diseases of the body that cause a lot of psychic problems such as those seen with Parkinson's disease, multiple sclerosis, paraneoplastic syndromes, dementia.

Rather than adopting these disease models, Bion (1977) took a different and interesting approach in using the analogy of Picasso's glass painting, a painting which is visible on both sides of the glass plate. In Bion's use of this as a metaphor, one side is the psyche interpreting unrepresented messages of the body, for instance in dreams. The other side of the glass painting stands for the body that interprets what happens in the psyche but in its own bodily language (for instance by the gut brain, heart brain, immune system...). Besides this metaphor of the glass painting, we may also represent the relationship between psyche and body as a kind of screen on which shadows are projected, from both the psychic and the somatic sides.

These models correspond with the work of the neuroscientist Ledoux. In Ledoux, 2015, he stated that his former theory of the emotional brain

(Ledoux, 1998) was wrong but despite recanting it his 1998 emotional brain theory is still the reigning paradigm in our psychoanalytic field. According to his 1998 theory, a perception evokes an emotional reaction in the basic brain (amygdala-thalamus) which then gets elaborated in the cognitive cortical brain. But in 2015 he changed his ideas and his current theory is more a kind of dual track system, in which some reactions happen at a psychic level—while other reactions remain in the body. This latter model allows for two different pathways that are not necessarily linked with each other. This dual track point of view may have large consequences for psychoanalysis and psychotherapy in general—but especially for the treatment of trauma and psychosomatic problems. It means that we need to reach the patient not only at the mentalizing (Transformation in K level or second zone) but also at the experiencing "bodymind" (Transformation in O or third zone) level.

Psychosomatic psychoanalysis

Likewise, the challenge of making contact with both the mind and the "bodymind" is reflected in the psychoanalytic approach toward (psycho) somatic diseases. The French psychosomatic school with Marty (1980), Luquet, and Aisenstein has probably the greatest tradition in working with somatic and psychosomatic illnesses. The French School developed a model that basically focused on "mentalization", corresponding to the second zone in the zonal model. It can be seen as emphasizing "symbolization"—psychic elaboration of inner impulses, drives. In psychosomatic patients they found "a pensée opératoire", an "operative thinking" with a lack of psychic elaboration. It is not unlike the "alexithymia" of Sifneos (1972). The Paris School even developed a kind of scale to measure "mentalization" (which is different from what Fonagy et al. (1991) later called reflective functioning and mentalization). The focus of the Paris school is on developing "mentalization", or psychic processing of emotions (which corresponds to Bion's "thinking"). The Paris School has a tradition of research of this model. Translated to the "zonal" model proposed here, the Paris School approach focuses on the "second zone" of psychic functioning. Actually also in the Anglo-Saxon world most of the psychoanalytic approaches see a facilitation of the symbolizing, mentalizing activity as their main mechanism of change. This is also the case in the treatment of psychosis, autism, anorexia nervosa, trauma, and borderline conditions.

Following Bion's distinction of the psychosomatic and the somatopsychic realm, this mentalizing approach is probably only one leg of the treatment in severe pathology, trauma, and somatic problems—the second zone. What about the other leg of treatment?

We may find an answer to this question in the work of Jacques Press (2015, 2019) of the Swiss Psychoanalytical Society, an answer that proposes a quite different move in the approach to psychosomatic problems. Press advocates an approach which recognizes the importance of "l'insuffisance de l'âme" (the insufficiency of the soul) and attempts contact with undifferentiated psychic functioning. Being in contact with this undifferentiated world has a freeing—healing effect. The work of Press is mainly influenced by Winnicott's ideas on regression to formlessness. From a Winnicottian point of view, the undifferentiatedness of the "in-between mind" which is imbedded in the psychesoma has an effect on the body.

Translated to the zonal model, it can be stated that by faults and insufficiency in the second zone, contact with the third zone can be facilitated. At this level of undifferentiatedness there is no longer any difference between body and mind.

How can we be in contact with the third zone and reach the real body (das Leib) in psychoanalysis?

The dual track model of Ledoux implies that functioning in the second and the third zone happens separately and in parallel but that changes in the third zone may occasionally get to the second zone and get represented there. The second zone is the zone where the symbolizing and mentalizing of emotional experiences occurs. Any effects on the real or BHSGIbody, as it is called in this paper, happen through activity in the third zone, which is undifferentiated, unrepresentable, and unknowable.

Psychoanalysis can have a direct effect on the third zone (even without being noticed by patient and/or analyst) and can facilitate the flow from the third to the second zone (O to K). However, the third zone cannot be reached through second zone activity like reverie (in Bion's terms we cannot go from K to O), or first zone activity (Reason).

A direct contact with the third zone in a verbal therapy may for instance happen through the frame, the psychoanalytic device in which the rhythm of the sessions, the room, the smell, the voice, are important as a background. This "background" is not experienced at the level of Reasoning or at a reverie-imaginary level, but rather is experienced at an undifferentiated level of which the patient is not always aware. This non-verbal background is so important in some patients that it can be called a "background mother" (Vermote, 2019c).

A decrease of the second zone activity is necessary to facilitate the flow from the third to the second zone. The way that Bion proposed facilitating this movement, is by giving no food to the second zone through his technique of "no memory, no desire, no senses, no coherence". No judging and no understanding are part of it as well. Metaphorically speaking, this corresponds to a movement downward in the second zone, attempting to be as close as possible to the infinity of the third zone. Bion advised analyzing as close to infinity as possible. This is not unlike the Japanese Mu-shin (Nishihira & Matsuki, 2017) or Chinese Wu-shin. This attitude corresponds to a maximal containment, a containment in emptiness, a kind of "non-containment containment" (Vermote, 2020).

It also corresponds to Bion's (1970) psychoanalytic attitude of an Act of Faith, which is opposite to an attitude from a K dimension (or second zone). Moreover, from being close to the third infinite zone, talking becomes a "language of Achievement". There is no more difference, but instead undifferentiatedness and therefore a becoming. This language of Achievement may have many aspects of the deeper unconscious layers of the second zone that may be reflected in primary process characteristics.

Other ways of decreasing second zone activity outside of psychoanalysis, are for instance by losing oneself in art, sports, love, religion, and by the experience of the "Sublime" where the second zone is overwhelmed. Meditation and hallucinogenic drugs may also have this effect on the second zone.

It is striking that in *Cured*, J. Rediger (2021) researched in a retrospective, qualitative way what happened in patients with incurable diseases like a neuroglioblastoma who experienced an unexplained, spontaneous healing process. He looked for patterns (like diet, way of living, dealing with the disease, and so on.) and finally came to two main hypothetical factors: belief and what he called a decrease of the DMN. Belief is an Act of Faith, a third zone activity and a decrease of DMN, and consequently it means a decrease of second zone activity.

This corresponds to the final lines of Bion's (1970) last theoretical book, *Attention and Interpretation*.

In these final lines Bion writes:

> what is to be sought is an activity that is both the restoration of god (the Mother) and the evolution of god (the formless, infinite, ineffable, non-existent), which can be found only in a state in which there is NO memory, desire, understanding.
>
> (Bion, 1970, p. 129)

This somewhat enigmatic message about the essence of psychoanalysis means: the restoration of god-Mother is the restoration of the primary-sensation mother (the background mother, third zone); the evolution of god is an evolution of an unknowable, non-verbal, formless, and unrepresentable infinite world (third zone) which can happen when the analyst diminishes K or second zone activity.

A clinical case fragment, as a kind of illustration of this approach (not a proof)

D is a lady in her forties. We worked through internal patterns and phantasies governing her relationships. When the ending of the analysis arrived as a topic, something happened at a different level from the free associations: she started losing all her hair. Her body reacted violently, but this happened outside and independent of verbal thinking. Falling back on the safety of the sessions (what is called the background mother in the text above), the physical process stopped, and her hair recovered. Further contact with the undifferentiated third zone happened in an unexpected way. The patient was always graciously dressed up to attend her sessions and I did not know her otherwise. One day, by intuition I saw her as if she were imprisoned. In her associations that followed, it became clear that her dressing up was not agreeable, but driven by a meticulous, demanding schedule. She had to visit her ill mother, had to be on time for a partial job, shop for groceries, and participate in sports. Even when she had a shortage of time, she felt she needed to follow her schedule and even go home before the session to change her clothes. If she failed, she felt like she was being sucked in by a big black hole, which she compared to a cladding of black ink that was spreading. The only way to combat this feeling was to follow her demanding schedule. This could sooth the terror of a hole in her mental functioning (or second zone functioning in the presented model). Once this phenomenon was revealed, it was clear that there was more at play than a reflection of her separation anxiety and archaic super-ego, as I had treated it before. There was a kind of madness to it, that Press (2015) would call a blank obsession, without content, which is often seen in psychosomatic patients, as well as in cases of substance abuse and can also be the drive behind frenetic work or creativity. So far, I had worked by giving second zone reverie-based interventions, which soothed her. It had been about separation anxiety and an archaic super-ego. But now, I saw a kind of madness too, a blank obsession. Instead of giving interventions that gave food to the second zone and soothed her, I saw what was happening as an opportunity to be in contact with the third zone and so I reacted instead with an "act of Faith". In nothingness, my shift in listening and intervening had an effect of relaxing her and led to decreasing her frenetic activity, her usual defensive behavior. This containment by nothingness was a new experience. "Losing herself" was actually not leading to a fragmented self, but to a better and freer functioning of the second zone. The fear of being clad in spreading black ink changed by moments into more peaceful feelings of emptiness. Her free associations took place against another background, a background of the primary-sensation mother.

Conclusion

This text discusses the difficult problem of the body-mind interaction from a Bionian point of view. An integrative model, mainly based on Bion's ideas of psychic functioning, is presented. This model offers conceptual support for working closely with the ineffable, undifferentiated fields of the "body-mind". Some implications for psychoanalytic technique are mentioned.

References

Bion, W.R. (1961). *Experiences in groups.* Tavistock.

Bion, W.R. (1962). A theory of thinking. In W.R. Bion (1967), *Second thoughts*. Jason Aronson.

Bion, W.R. (1970). *Attention and interpretation*. Karnac.

Bion, W.R. (1977/1991). *A memoir of the future*. Karnac.

Carhart-Harris, R.L., & Friston, K.J. (2010). The default-mode, ego-functions and free-energy: a neurobiological account of Freudian ideas. *Brain*, 133, 1265–1283.

Fonagy, P. (1991). Thinking about thinking: Some clinical and theoretical considerations in the treatment of a borderline patient. *International Journal of Psychoanalysis*, 72, 639–656.

Freud, S. (1915). The Unconscious. In *The standard edition of the complete psychological works of Sigmund Freud* (Vol. XIV).

Freud, S. (1933). New introductory lectures on psycho-analysis and other works. In *The standard edition of the complete psychological works of Sigmund Freud* (Vol. XXII).

Grotstein, J.S. (2007). *A beam of intense darkness*. Karnac.

Klein, M. (1935). A contribution to the psychogenesis of manic-depressive states. *Int. J. Psycho-Anal.*, 16, 145–174.

Klein, M. (1946). Notes on some schizoid mechanisms. *Int. J. Psycho-Anal.*, 27, 99–110.

Ledoux, J. (1998). *The emotional brain*. Simon and Schuster.

Ledoux, J. (2015). *Anxious: Using the brain to understand and treat fear and anxiety*. Viking.

Nishihira, T., & Matsuki, K. (2017). *Mu-shin no Taiwa (Dialogue of Mind-No Mind)*. Sogensha.

Marty, P. (1980). *L'Ordre psychosomatique*. Payot.

Mason, M.F., et al. (2007). Wandering minds: The default network and stimulus-independent thought. *Science*, 315(5810), 393–395.

Matte Blanco, I. (1988). *Thinking, feeling and being: Clinical reflections on the fundamental antinomy of human beings*. Routledge.

Press, J. (2015). Le transfer du négatif. Histoire d'une possession blanche. *Revue Française de Psychanalyse*, 4(79).

Press, J. (2019). Le psychanalyste et le psychésoma. Transformer le destin en destinée, un enjeu psychosomatique. *Revue française de psychosomatique*, 56, 93–103.

Rediger, J. (2021). *Cured. The power of our immune system and the mind-body connection*. Penguin Books.

Sifneos, P.E. (1972). The prevalence of 'alexithymic' characteristics in psychosomatic patients. *Psychotherapy and Psychosomatics*, 22(2), 255–262.

Vermote, R. (2013). The undifferentiated zone of psychic functioning: An integrative approach and clinical implications. *Bulletin of the European Federation of Psychoanalysis*, 13, 16–27.

Vermote, R. (2014). Transformations et transmissions du fonctionnement psychique: Approche integrative et implications cliniques. *Revue française de psychanalyse*, LXXVIII(2), 389–405.

Vermote, R. (2019a). *Reading Bion: a chronological exploration of Bions writings*. The New Library of Psychoanalysis Teaching Series. Routledge.

Vermote, R. (2019b). *Different mind-body relationships at different levels of psychic functioning, from a Bionian point of view*. Panel notes on the body in the theories of Freud, Winnicott and Bion, Panel Conference of the European Federation of

Psychoanalysis, Jasminka Šuljagić, Rudi Vermote, and Jan Abram, Madrid, 12 April 2019.

Vermote, R. (2019c). *Trauma and primal repression.* Lecture, British Society of Psychoanalysis, London, March 2019.

Vermote, R. (2020). Psychic functioning outside of mental representations. Implications for psychoanalysis. *The Journal of the Japan Psychoanalytic Society,* 20(2), 3–16.

Winnicott, D.W. (1949). Mind and its relation with psyche-soma. In *Collected works* (Vol. 3).

Chapter 6

Being totally in the dark

On working analytically within the depths of the great unknown of psychic catastrophe

Ofra Eshel

Contemporary psychoanalytic approaches strive to extend the reach of psychoanalytic treatment to more and most disturbed patients, to more deeply disturbed aspects of patients' personalities and experiences, to difficult treatment situations, and deep non-communicating layers.

Over the past decades, psychoanalytic thinking has moved theoretically and clinically to the realms of trauma, both personal and general, direct or transmitted across generations, and to emphasizing the "distortion of essential processes that are basic to object-relating" (Winnicott, 1963, p. 180). This has called for changes in psychoanalytic thinking and technique. Working psychoanalytically with non-neurotic patients and states of mind challenges traditional theory and practice, and, in my opinion, forges an emerging dimension of presence and analytic oneness that 21st-century psychoanalysis is not only moving toward but must also deepen into in order to cope with its clinical challenges.

This move also resonates with the ontological shift currently taking place in psychoanalysis (Eshel, 2004, 2017a, 2019a; Ogden, 2019), which reflects a fundamental commitment to the principle of *being and becoming in the experience* rather than epistemological exploration and interpretation.

Being-with and transformations in oneness

For many years, from the beginning of my therapeutic work with patients and especially during my years as an analyst, I have been intrigued by the complex, difficult, and gripping nature of the analytic work; the ways it is (re) created and found, again and again, in each psychoanalytic endeavor and patient-analyst encounter—particular and unique, often unexpected and unknown, and sometimes even mysterious.

Based on this clinical experience, the two key ideas which over the years have crystalized and developed into my own way of psychoanalytic thinking and working, are the analyst/therapist's "presencing" (being-there) within the patient's experiential psychic reality and within the grip of the analytic process, and the ensuing patient-analyst experiential-emotional interconnectedness or

DOI: 10.4324/9781003534365-6

"withnessing"—thus forging an emergent new entity of patient-with-analyst, *a two-in-oneness*, that may deepen into *at-one-ment* with the patient's innermost emotional reality. Analyst and patient are inevitably bound together through this way of analytic work. This is primarily an *interconnected* relatedness rather than an interactive relationship, and it concentrates on the *ontological (being) quality* of the analytic experience that is lived through *with* the analyst rather than the epistemological (knowing) and interpretive qualities. The analyst gives himself over to becoming part of the patient's ongoing emotional reality and mental processes. Patient and analyst "*live an experience together*" (Winnicott 1945, p. 152, italics in original; see also Ogden, 2001), or they "live the unthinkable, the unexperienced, and the unlived t(w)ogether" in living through extremely dark, unknown processes in difficult treatments (Eshel, 2019b). I have also called this process in its extreme singularity "quantum interconnectedness" (from physicist David Bohm's [1980] phrase "the quantum interconnectedness of distant systems"), in order to convey the profound implications of this quantum-like psychoanalytic quality of experience.[1]

The spectrum of analytic oneness

This way of working is a fundamental dimension of my analytic work with patients. But varying states of the unknown or unthought intensify and develop into the full need and the full potential the ways of being-, becoming-, and experiencing-in-oneness in the analytic work; namely, the analytic oneness as an essential resource for the process of transformation.

In this regard, Vermote's (2013) model of psychic functioning for dealing with the unthought in psychoanalytic work, identifies three distinct zones or modes of psychic functioning with various degrees of differentiation, different psychoanalytic models, and clinical implications for the analyst:

1. Reason—oedipal, understanding Ucs. system (Freud, Klein)

2. Transformations in Knowledge—container-contained, reverie, dream-work, alpha function (Bion, Ogden, Ferro, Marty, de M'Uzan, Botella and Botella, Bollas).

3. Transformations in O, when dealing with the most unthought, unknown, undifferentiated mode of psychic functioning (Winnicott, Milner, late Bion, late Lacan). Profound psychic *change* with life-giving quality occurs *at the level of radical experience, unrepresented and* unknowable-O (called O by Bion for Origin),[2] while the *epistemological exploration* of the traumatic unknown, in mode 2 of transformation in Knowledge or dream-thought, remains at the level of representations. Thus, the difference between *transformation in Knowledge* and *transformation in O* is that T(K) is a thought for something that has not been thought yet, and T(O) is a new experience that happens, that "becomes" at a non-differentiated level within the transference (Vermote, 2013).

I have further proposed a *spectrum of analytic oneness*—a spectrum of varying degrees of analytic oneness within different unconscious or unknown states and non-communicating layers in the analytic work. It focuses primarily on the extent of the traumatization or the distortion of fundamental processes of relatedness and the incapacity to represent, which is disrupted, regressively lost, or failed to develop. At the same time, it opens up new ontological-experiential (versus epistemological) possibilities for working within difficult psychic realities:

I. The Freudian repressed unconscious—consists of psychic material that could have been repressed, in which *"the interpretation of dreams is the royal road to a knowledge of the unconscious activities of the mind"* (Freud, 1900, p. 608, italics in original); that is, an epistemological exploration for the recovering of repressed material through the interpretation and analysis of the transference and the interpretation of dreams. This is the most differentiated mode of analytic functioning.

However, despite the centrality of the Freudian repressed unconscious, Freud himself (1915, 1923) pointed out that although what is repressed is unconscious, the unconscious is not only the repressed:

> We recognize that the *Ucs.* does not coincide with the repressed; it is still true that all that is repressed is *Ucs.*, but not all that is *Ucs.* is repressed. … we find ourselves thus confronted by the necessity of postulating a third *Ucs.*, which is not repressed.
>
> (1923, p. 18, italics in the original)

II. The unrepressed unconscious of non-neurotic patients and states of mind, consists of psychic material that could not be repressed, but is dissociated, split-off, and may become unrepresented (Levine et al., 2013; Vermote, 2013; Bergstein, 2014; Eshel, 2017a, 2019a). Thus, the unconscious in the realms of unbearable and catastrophic psychic trauma is no longer the repressed unconscious of psychoneurosis. It is the unrepressed unconscious, and it attempts to extend psychoanalytic practice beyond psychoneurosis and beyond what were formerly thought to be the limits of analytic work (Levine, 2022). It ranges from the *unrepressed realm, level I*, that is traumatically dissociated and unknown, to the deeper *unrepressed and unrepresented realm, levelII,* of the most unknown and unknowable, unthinkable psychic reality; the deepest traumatic and non-communicating issues of human life.

Analytic work in the unrepressed unconscious entails being in various degrees of patient-and-analyst state of oneness and transformations in oneness, moving from patient-and-analyst *two-in-oneness* to *at-one-ment* with the patient's unrepressed and unrepresented psychic reality:

Level I. The unbearable traumatic unknown remains at the level of partial or weak representations—"was it or was it not" and "shadows" of remembering (Eshel & Zeligman, 2017)—and can be transformed by analytic representations through the analyst's reverie, dream-thought, alpha function, containing capacity in Bionian, intersubjective, and analytic field models; and "vicarious introspection" in Kohut's Self psychology—these are "transformations in K" (Bion, 1967, 1970; Vermote, 2013); thus transforming t(w)ogether, even as one mind dissociates, through *patient-with-analyst two-in-oneness.*

Level II. But in the most unfathomable and unthinkable realm of traumatization that the psyche could not bear, in particular the great unknown of mental catastrophe (Bion, 1970) and early breakdown (Winnicott, 1974, 1965), the patient's emotional reality is mostly unthinkable, unexperienced, unrepressed, and unrepresented. This necessitates going *beyond* the limits of representations and analytic thinking, dreaming and containing (K) to terms of *being*—to the ontological-experiential analytic work of being-there (presencing), with-in the innermost emotional reality of the trauma, becoming at-one-with[3] the patient's most traumatic psychic reality. *Thus,* the depths of the unknown, especially the most traumatic unknown, where the patient's emotional reality is mostly unthinkable, unexperienced, and unrepresented, necessitate—by definition—going beyond epistemological exploration to the analytic work of being and becoming with-in the patient's psychic reality, at-one-with the patient's innermost emotional reality. *The unthinkable cannot be thought, but only relived and gone through with or at-one-with the analyst.*

In the grip of the unknown

From this broader and basic introductory context, I will proceed to the subject of this chapter—working analytically within the depths of the great unknown of psychic catastrophe.

The clinical example that I have chosen to illustrate the work of experiencing, being, and becoming with-in the patient's unknown realms of emotional catastrophe, is an extreme example (published previously, 2001, 2019a). It describes my experience of sleeping during treatment. I chose it because this treatment made me go through and face, more so than any other clinical example that I have written about, an experience that deeply puzzled me. When I first wrote about it, more than twenty years ago, I focused primarily on the subject of the analyst's 'sleep'. I reviewed the psychoanalytic literature on the analyst's sleeping during sessions, and then focused on exploring my own sleeping and its qualities of experience while also relating to the deliberation over self-exposure and concealment of such experiences. In 2019b, I added in this regard Bion's (2005) powerful words in his sixth Rome seminar (on 16 July 1977—Morning), at the age of eighty:

> It seems to me that the analyst who actually participates in the experience has a chance of deciding whether to try to communicate—as he is doing here—and whether we would be capable of hearing and understanding the communication. If he is to communicate the experience, which

language is he to talk? Will articulate speech do? ... In any case it requires courage if he is going to dare to make public, to communicate to somebody not himself, his experience. It may take a long time.

(p. 6)

In the present essay, I will focus mainly on the darkness and working totally in the dark, which resonates with Francesca Bion's description that Bion "often talked to her about his feelings of *being totally in the dark* ... He would say ... 'It's beyond me', or, 'I can't make head or tail of it'" (1995/2014, p. 96, my italics). These words strongly express my overwhelming experience during that analytic process.

I will first let the clinical material speak, describing a clinical sequence in which the extreme unknown during the sessions became an open issue, and closely follow my experience of being in the grip of this process as the treatment unfolded. I will then return to this dark unknown in the discussion, in an attempt to rethink and understand it more fully.

Clinical illustration

Background

Clari came to me unwillingly for treatment, after undergoing two years of twice-weekly face-to-face therapy with a female psychotherapist to whom she had become considerably attached. Clari, then in her early 30s, was born in South America, and was the second of three daughters born at three-year intervals. Her younger sister had been very ill from the age of six months. She was kept alive for nine years, in a permanent vegetative state, until her death when Clari was 12 years old, two years after the family immigrated to Israel, leaving the child behind in an institution. Clari married at 20, but her relationship with her husband was difficult and sexually frightening. She left him and, for nine years, lived with a woman in a stable but stagnant relationship dominated by her partner's obsessive-compulsive preoccupations. She originally sought therapy because of severe anxiety attacks during the Gulf War. The therapy was warm and supportive, in the best sense of the word, and led to a turnabout in her life: she decided she wanted to have children, but thought that children should grow up with a mother and a father. She therefore decided to leave the woman with whom she had been living and establish a relationship with a man.

It was at this point that Clari's psychotherapist was informed that, unexpectedly, she would be leaving Israel within a few months for family reasons. Therefore, she asked me to accept Clari for treatment, as she was concerned about abandoning her at such a stage of critical decision-making. I was unable to accept Clari then, since I had no vacancy, and suggested referring her to another therapist, but Clari's psychotherapist pressed me to take her because she felt I was strong enough to treat Clari during this angry, stormy time. I finally agreed, on the condition that the treatment begin in six months' time.

Before committing ourselves to treatment, Clari and I met once, at her suggestion. During that session, she expressed a reluctant and rejecting attitude toward me, glancing suspiciously at the couch—even though she would be coming for twice-weekly face-to-face therapy, as in the therapy she had been undergoing—saying that she would never have gone to a psychoanalyst for treatment, and the only reason that she came was because her therapist had recommended me so warmly. I said only that I understood it was hard to change treatment in this way. At the end of the session, after Clari checked that I had no long-term plans to leave the country over the next few years, we set a date for starting treatment.

When Clari came in to start treatment, she appeared lost and depressed, unlike how she appeared at our first meeting. Over the previous few months, she had been very lonely, both because her therapy had ended and because her relationship with her woman friend had ended, and her friend had already formed a new relationship with another woman. She calmed down soon after treatment began, and it became apparent that the fact that treatment was taking place made her feel more held.

During the first two years of treatment that followed, she was very lonely, cut off from her former circle of women (lesbian) friends, yet resolute in her decision to establish a serious relationship with a man. Little by little, she told me that she had been repeatedly dreaming what she called "dreams of force"—horrific dreams she had had before but which were now recurring with increasing frequency. In these dreams she was always in the familiar surroundings of her home and bedroom, when suddenly, everything would go dark, with an overpowering, sinister feeling of terror. She would usually try to do something—get up, switch on the light—without success, becoming slower, paralyzed. Then she would be gripped and overcome by a tremendous force exerting a terrible, crushing pressure on her chest and especially on her head, and she would be unable to move. She knew that there was no point in struggling; all she could do was submit and lie still until it passed, so that it would spare her and not kill her, and try to just continue breathing—to just survive.[4]

Despite sleeping very lightly, she could not avoid the dreams, which occurred even when she slept during the day. But gradually, over the first two years of treatment with me, the frequency of the dreams decreased, and her numerous physical pains also diminished. Clari settled into a new job and studies, and in the third year of treatment, after unsuccessfully dating several men, her relationship with her estranged husband, who over the years would phone her once a year on her birthday, was slowly and cautiously renewed. They experienced many difficulties at first; each time they quarreled she would become frightened and threaten to end the relationship. They again encountered sexual problems, but her husband, who over the years had undergone psychotherapy, was given great, direct encouragement by his therapist to persevere in the relationship, and he showed a determination and patience that he had not had in previous years. The relationship stabilized, and they moved in together, hoping to start a family.

The zone of darkness

In moving from the description of the *events* in Clari's treatment to the treatment itself and the quality and texture of the therapeutic relationship, I enter another realm, opaque and shadowy—a zone of darkness.

From our first session in treatment, Clari spoke in a manner that was spare, restrained, vague, unclear—it is difficult for me even to find the word that might precisely describe the way she spoke. Often, I could not hear or understand what she was saying. Initially, I thought and interpreted that she found it difficult to talk to me because she had come to me for treatment against her will (and, in fact, against mine, too); but as treatment continued, there was no change. Later on, I thought that perhaps she was afraid of evolving erotic transference, or that I was afraid of it, but I quickly realized that these were rather simplistic, external interpretations. Something was strangling her capacity to communicate, but what was it?

She seemed just to need my presence there. She attended treatment regularly, never missing a session or arriving late. At the beginning of the session she would examine me closely, and then begin talking in her vague, stiff, disconnected way, her face immobile. After ten or fifteen minutes, my laborious attentiveness would gradually diminish, and I would become detached. It was not that my thoughts wandered or that I was bored. Nothing. Blank. Absent. I ceased to exist as a person who listened, thought, and responded. I would sometimes become numb and sleepy. Then, in the last ten minutes of the session, I would come out of it and become myself again, listening, relating, responding.

This pattern bore little relation to my feelings of fatigue. While at the beginning fatigue would hasten the process, later on it made no real difference.

By the beginning of the fourth year of treatment, after the decisions and changes described earlier in Clari's life had been discussed in the treatment and actually made, and were thus less central to the therapeutic discourse, this situation became particularly acute, so that after the first ten to fifteen minutes of listening and responding, I would fall into a deep sleep, totally devoid of feeling. Then, in the last ten minutes, I would wake up. This was all while sitting facing her, thus I was unable to conceal it and, in fact, I did not try to.

When I first began falling asleep, Clari was very surprised that I dared close my eyes and be with her in a situation in which I was "so very unprotected and exposed". She repeatedly said that even with her woman friend, during their long relationship, over all the years of knowing each other and living together, neither ever closed her eyes in the presence of the other, not even during their intimate games and sex, because they were afraid of each other. She said that her woman friend would say that she was afraid of a streak of cold cruelty in Clari. Clari herself never dared fall soundly sleep. "As far back as I can remember, I would never sleep at night", she said.

She then began to fear that I would decide to terminate the treatment because of what was happening. Thereupon I told her that, *indeed, something very strange was happening to me, and I could only suggest that we let things be until we could better understand what was going on.* (This was what I truly thought and felt.) Clari was silent for a moment, and then said, "All right", in a voice I could barely hear, and she appeared very pensive and far less tense; her entire body seemed to relax. Much later she would tell me that, throughout this entire period, up until I said this, she had been terrified that "the situation would become so unbearable that you would be unable to endure it, that you would stop breathing or stop the treatment, or that I would go mad." She was convinced that I was about to tell her that after trying years of treatment with her, it was clear that there was no point in continuing, and that she should see another therapist. She would not be able to argue with this, as it was completely logical, but for her, it would be fatal. In her own words, "Then all is lost. We won't be saved. Death." (This, however, was only said to me much later—after shifting from psychotherapy to analysis.)

But, at this stage, things continued in the same way for several months, and my direct efforts to understand my recurring sleeping, to discuss and consult, were to no avail. I examined various ideas, but felt unable to really understand or change it. I did not seem to have an inner clue for comprehending what was happening to me. My only feeling was that of a massive sinking into sleep, without emotions, without understanding, without thoughts (at the time, I didn't even ask myself or Clari what was happening to her while I was asleep). It was like something extremely dissociative, or like being under anesthesia after receiving a sleep-inducing injection. I therefore felt that I could only rely on the truth and the necessity of the treatment process, on its hidden meaning and order, and on its own reality. So I let things be and waited to see what would evolve.

This continued until one session, while still in this deep sleep, I saw a kind of schematic drawing of a bright tunnel with a small black dot moving up and down in its center. That was the first time that I saw or felt something while in this state, and I awoke with an unfamiliar sense of relief.

When Clari came to the following session, she was extremely troubled, sitting pale and silent. I waited and then remarked that she seemed troubled. She said, "No", probably because she thought I was referring to her reaction to my recurring sleeping, "Your tiredness is sometimes hard for me, but *after last time,* I thought that we are both stubborn, and when one of us weakens, the other keeps holding, and vice versa". "Yes", I said, and she gave a faint smile of relief. She fell silent again, very much within herself, and then said that she had dreamt a dream or, perhaps, hadn't dreamt at all. Perhaps it had been a kind of fantasy or a memory-scene.

> *It was dark, she got up to pee, and then she saw this scene. She heard someone shouting, "No, no, no, no", a terrible cry, and she suddenly understood that it was her. Then she saw a baby, swollen from beatings, being put in a crib, a baby dressed in threadbare clothing, looking like a corpse. She saw the shadow of the person who was laying the baby down, perhaps the shadow of a woman, and she, as a little girl, was climbing up the crib's rail to see.*

This profoundly frightened her. *Who was it? Was it memory or fantasy?* It had seemed so very real — "no feeling of a dream." Was the baby her sister, who at the age of six months had become a vegetable, who would lie in bed, hooked up to feeding tubes because she didn't eat? Had something happened to her? But her mother had said that even earlier she felt there was something wrong with the baby, and had taken her to all kinds of doctors. Since her sister was three years younger than she was, it seemed to fit the dream … was she herself the baby? There were the threadbare clothes, white trousers, a flannel shirt. She used to wear shabby clothes … there was an orphanage near their home, so perhaps it was something she saw there (Clari's speech was very fragmented). But, if it were her, how was she able to see it all? It was like a split within her. This frightened her greatly. She was unable to go back to sleep. She thought that this memory—the horribly battered baby—explained all the pain and the terrible somatic things she had experienced in the past: the pains in her arms and hands, the illnesses at the beginning of her marriage, the other terrible pains. Her whole body had been sick and in pain for years.

The next time she dreamt, it was again a dream of darkness, as though darkness had had erupted and taken over her entire world:

> *I am outside, in the neighborhood, in a park, and suddenly it turns dark. A feeling of a power failure, and then a light failure. I can't see a thing, there's this total darkness, with no stars, no light at all. I tell myself I must go home, but it's impossible even to know which way to go, because everything is so terribly dark. There is a feeling that something dangerous is about to happen, something evil … and I woke up terrified, my heart pounding wildly. Darkness like the darkness before I saw the scene of the baby, like in the dream of force.*
>
> *It's obvious that the darkness is an omen of bad things to come. I have to remind myself that there is life, because in some strange way, if I don't remember, if I don't hold on to reality, I'll become smaller and smaller and*

disappear into something like that, something dark, and empty, and suffo-
cating. I think that the baby in the dream is me. That explains a lot of
things, all the terrible somatic things. When I tell myself this, it's with a
horrific feeling, of death, because it was dying, and then to live, you have to
hold on to having to breathe, otherwise you'll stop. Living. Just to go on
breathing. A sensation that gives me the feeling it could be reality. Not
even panic, not to move, just being aware of having to breathe.

Dreams and dream-thoughts

In the period that followed, her dreams, their images, the experiences they
expressed and their sequence enabled us to get into and explore the ongoing
brutal seesawing between holding and falling, hope and destruction; to
recognize Clari's longing and struggle to work her way toward feeling that
trust was a valid response to catastrophe. For the first time, she began
dreaming different dreams, dreams of hope, of being helped and of a helping
figure. And then, in the nights that immediately followed, again, unbearable
dreams, with scenes of horror and disaster. In the first different, new dream,

She goes to sleep, and in their bedroom, there is a little girl of about three,
curled up and dressed only in panties. She [Clari] gets up, because she
understands that if she doesn't take care of the child, no one will. She takes
the child's hand and leads her into a room of her own—all is very dark, a
wind is blowing and the curtains flying—and she dresses her in a night-
gown. The child is happy, gets into bed, and before she falls asleep says, "I
thought the whole house was going to collapse, but it's only Grandma who
died."

Clari was deeply moved and fought back tears—which appeared for
the first time during the treatment—when we talked about the dream.
"My feeling is always kind of hazy. I have a lot of stumps", she said. "All
of life is built on something that isn't there. It's like in movie cartoons—
you keep going on nothing, you look down and then you see that the
ground isn't there, that you've been running on air."

Yet, each hopeful dream was immediately followed by dreams of catastrophe in which hope, change, prospects, and her sleep were attacked
and shattered—although in these dreams, too, amid the shattering, now
there were the beginnings of struggles for help, either in the dream, or in
the waking up that followed it. The night after telling me the preceding
hopeful dream, Clari was thrown back into a harrowing "dream of
force", in which she was in bed, and a sensation of paralysis and pressure
began, particularly in her head, which was big, swollen, and heavy. She
got up to turn on the light, and there was no electricity. Horrified, she
tried over and over to turn on other lights, with no success, her entire
body gradually becoming incapable of movement. She woke up confused

and disorientated. The sensation continued for a long time; she didn't know who she was. She said to me,

I remembered you before I remembered me. And then I said to you, to me, "Just a second, I'm Clari, I'm 35 years old. There's Ron [her husband]". And then I told myself where I am in my life, where I work, and where I live. I almost called to tell you that something evil was about to happen, and then I realized that it wasn't real. But the sensation and the swelling in my head continued. I felt a need to eat, and I sat down and ate.

In another disastrous dream, the little girl from the previous hopeful dream was drowning, as though the good dream could not be supported for long—

Clari is with her husband and the little girl near a water reservoir, and the girl falls into the water. And when she falls in, she stops breathing, doesn't do a thing, curls up, and begins to sink ... the water is very deep. Clari yells to her husband to jump in and save her because the girl isn't breathing, isn't breathing. Ron begins undressing to jump into the water but has problems with his laces, and then she jumps into the water with her clothes on and begins to dive deeper underwater, but she cannot reach the little girl because the reservoir is very deep. She comes up for air and tries to dive down again, but it is clear to her that she cannot save the child. She thinks: Why doesn't Ron jump in, maybe he can reach her. *It's not clear whether he jumped in or not.*

Again, the agonizing inability to be saved and to save, although there was a desperate attempt by Clari at saving.

Were the dreams heading toward a null point, a breakdown, the collapse of a new beginning?

On the threshold of analysis: Between the darkness and the dread to know

Two months after the scene of the mortally battered baby, Clari asked to switch to analysis. She said she felt that she "needed to be in more treatment at this time". I agreed, but would only be able to begin analysis six months later.

Then, in the following session, a very significant one, there was a recurrence of my massive falling asleep. Clari began the session by saying, "Now that we like each other more"—I was surprised because she had never previously used any words expressing such feelings—"I want to tell you something else". She told me that when she was a little girl, she felt she was a boy, a hyperactive boy; she would go to the bathroom and pee through a tube. She never told this to anyone, but there was something very confused in her, causing her learning difficulties and memory problems in school in spite of her great efforts at studying. I heard her up to this point, and then I fell into a deep sleep, awaking for the last ten minutes of the session. Clari said that she was observing me "from outside", as though she were seeing the little girl sinking in the dream, as though she were seeing herself as a boy. This boy had been there since she was three years old, since nursery school. When they hit her, he was strong, so they couldn't trample her.

There was something so palpable in her words that I found myself asking, "And what was his name?"

"Johnny," she said.

I said, "You needed trust to tell me this." Apparently, I had said too much.

Clari shrank back and responded cuttingly, "Trust is needed to be here for such a long time while you sleep." She was silent; then she said, "Yes, I really never, ever told anyone about him, ever."

From this point on, she began to sleep more soundly at night, and I, during the sessions, was becoming less and less sleepy; maybe it began before, but now it was clear. The mixture of good and terrifying dreams continued, but these were dreams with a frightening content and no longer "dreams of force" in which "there is only sensation; no content." She said, "There's no getting out of a dream of force. I'm in it; it's a horror that I can't even think. But now, when the anxiety overwhelms me, I think and come out of it".

In addition, she would now scream in her sleep, out of the terror of the frightening dreams, screaming for help. Even when her mouth was paralyzed and only sounds emanated, her husband would hear, wake up, and wake her. Now there was a scream and there was someone who heard.

Then there was another change. While on the border between sleep and wakefulness, she felt herself entering her own body, and it surrounded her like a thick, flexible, safe, protective tire, whereas previously she had observed her body and kept it protected from without.

She joined her mother on a family visit to the country of her birth, and there she went to the house where she had been born, but did not dare go inside. She also did not dare to sleep during the entire journey, until her return to Israel, and treatment.

On her return, strange, unknown details of her early childhood were suddenly revealed, following a question that she asked her parents about her childhood. Her father related that when Clari was six months old, her mother suddenly developed a strange illness that tests were unable to identify, "as though life seeped out of her." He took her to the maternal grandmother's house, and he returned home and to his work. The mother was put in the cellar, in the dark, while Clari was moved to the top floor. He said that her mother would constantly ask, "Where's Clari? Where's Clari?"

What went on there? Who looked after Clari? Where was the older sister? This all remained unfathomable, unresolved, and unanswered, flooded with fantasies. The conversation caused her mother and sister great anxiety, and it was impossible to ask any further questions.

At the end of these months, prior to the shift to analysis, Clari dreamt two dreams that strongly recapitulated the motifs of falling asleep, darkness, and terror. I will conclude the clinical illustration by describing them in Clari's own words.

The first dream took place before I left for a month-long vacation, some two months before the shift to analysis; in it there was a close connection between her being able to fall asleep, despite the dark, in face-to-face togetherness with me, and her capacity for separating afterwards.

> *It is terribly dark in here. I am lying on the couch, covered with a blanket from home, and you are sitting on a chair next to me, and then at some point you think I've fallen asleep, and you slowly get onto the couch and cover yourself. We are both lying on our sides, face-to-face, and then, in that position, I really do fall asleep, until at some point you wake me, and you're in a hurry, you have to leave, and there are all kinds of things that I dropped that you give me—car keys, my earrings, and some other things. We leave and you turn right, assuming that I'm going with you. There's a big parking lot there, but I say, "No, no, I parked on the left", and then we part.*

The second dream was just before the transition to analysis, after the session in which we finalized the two additional hours of analysis:

> *I am in my grandmother's house. The maid takes me into a room, the one that used to be mine, and when she switches on the light, the bulb burns out. It's a room that hasn't been used for a long time. She goes to get a bulb and leaves me in the dark, and I'm frightened. I ask her to take me first to the living room where everyone else is, but she already left. In the dark, I try to walk along the length of the wall, but I can't find the wall, as though there is a void all around; and yet I continue walking, with my arms out in front of me, searching for a wall, and the more I walk, the more frightening it becomes. I walk more and more slowly—these things from the dream of force, where everything begins to slow down. Eventually I can't move, I'm becoming paralyzed, with a feeling of approaching danger. By then I'm crawling and I open a door that I find. Apparently, it's the front door of the house. And then I'm even more terrified, because it's dark and I'm alone, and who knows who might come in, and I try to close the door and I can't, because I'm paralyzed. And I start to scream and scream from fear. And then someone comes in through the door, in a short skirt. She bends down and hugs me, and I see that it's my mother, and she's terribly upset, as though something very bad has happened, she's suffering a lot, and then she begins telling me that she wanted to tell the servants before she left that … and I wake myself up because I'm so terrified, so I don't have to hear. I know that there have been times in a dream when I woke myself up, so that I wouldn't hear something.*

I thought of her desperate struggle to break through the horrific, dark void and of the moment of the encounter she described in her dream. She had forged her way out from the horror of the darkness and the void-with-no-objects in which she was left alone, and from the grip of the paralysis, and finally reached her mother. But the mother, who could have contained and mitigated the horror, was herself very upset and overwhelmed (and over-whelming) by her own distress, and Clari fears knowing her. At the threshold of the door that she now opened, on the threshold of analysis, amid the des-perate helplessness, neediness, and the yearning to be helped, she fears that something unbearable has come in and will seize her through the contact with the motherly other.

Loneliness and longing, hope and dread (and the immense tension between them)—now, between the darkness and the dread to know, on the threshold of analysis...

Discussion

Darkness made visible

"If the analyst can take certain steps that enable him to 'see' what the patient sees, it is reasonable to suppose that the patient has likewise 'taken steps', though not necessarily the same ones, to enable him to 'see' what he sees", writes Bion (1970, p. 40).

The analyst's being- and becoming-with or at-one-with the patient's experiential reality which may enable him/her to "see" what the patient sees, is the essence of this discussion—"Darkness made visible."

"Darkness made visible" are words related to astrophysics. Almost 27 years ago, the metaphorical use of the astrophysical *"black hole"*, entered my psy-choanalytic thinking and writing (1998, 2017b, 2019a), and since then I have followed the developments in this area of astrophysics.

An astrophysical black hole is formed by the massive collapse of a dying star to a certain critical radius of infinitesimal size and almost infinite density ("singularity"), and its gravitational field becomes so strong that light can no longer escape—hence its blackness. In the years when Hawking and Gribbin wrote about the existence of "black holes" (Hawking, 1988, 1993; Gribbin, 1992), and when I first used metaphorically the astrophysical "black holes" in psychoanalysis (1998), there was no conclusive evidence from observation that black holes exist. Hawking himself expressed his concern about this:

> Black holes are one of only a fairly small number of cases in the history of science in which a theory was developed in great detail as a mathe-matical model before there was any direct evidence from observations that it was correct.... How could we hope to detect a black hole, as by its

very definition it does not emit any light? Fortunately, there is a way. ... a black hole exerts a gravitational force on nearby objects....

(1988, pp. 102–103).

Primordial black holes with masses more than a thousand million tons could be detected only by their gravitational *influence on other* visible matter or on the expansion of the universe.

(p. 108, my italics)

But during the next decades, astronomers and astrophysicists around the world have tried meticulously to provide visual evidence for the existence of black holes, despite the fact that the black hole itself cannot be seen because it is completely dark. In 2019 a global research team called the Event Horizon Telescope (EHT) Collaboration that turned the Earth into a giant receiver, released the first-ever image of a black hole—M87*, at the center of the Messier 87 galaxy, some 55 million light-years from Earth. This startling close-up image of a black hole's "shadow", showed a dark heart surrounded by a ring of light created by photons zipping around it. The evocative image was *Science*'s Breakthrough of the Year 2019: "Darkness made visible!"

On May 12, 2022, more than three years after the release of this first image of a black hole, scientists from the Event Horizon Telescope (EHT) have shared the stunning first image of Sagittarius A* (pronounced A-star)—the supermassive black hole lurking at the center of our own Milky Way galaxy. This image provides a long-anticipated look at the massive object that exists at the very center of our galaxy. Astronomers and astrophysicists had previously seen stars orbiting around something invisible, compact, and very massive at the center of the Milky Way. All this strongly suggested that this object—known as Sagittarius A* (Sgr A)—is a black hole, and the image provides the first direct visual evidence of it.

I would now like to address a similar process of transition from massive influence to making the darkness more visible and accessible in Clari's treatment. "Darkness" and "working totally in the dark" are used both figuratively and concretely in this account.

Clari's treatment confronted me with abysmal not-knowing and working totally in the dark, which profoundly resonated with Bion's words:

It means that I am forced to have an emotional experience and that I have to have it in such a way that I am unable to learn from it. I have consciousness, a sense organ enabling me to perceive the psychical qualities (as Freud puts it in The Interpretation of Dreams), but I am not to be allowed to comprehend it.

(1992, p. 220)

This necessitates working within the unthinkable and the unexperienced until *"the thing feared has been experienced"*, according to Winnicott's late clinical thinking (1974, 1965), or within something "more in the nature of a depersonalization or an extreme dissociation", as Winnicott refers to Scott's "regression to sleep" in Scott's presentation to the British Psycho-Analytical Society on January 27, 1954 (Winnicott, in Rodman, 1987, p. 56). For Bion, this is "a nameless dread" (1962) and the "dark night of/to the soul" (words borrowed from St. John of the Cross), which is the "'dark night' to K" in analytic work (1965, p.159). Described further in late Bion's powerful words, this is "a breakdown of dream-work-a" (1992, p. 59), "the complete dissociation" (2013, p. 68), "complete meaninglessness [when] all meaning, all source of meaning, has been annihilated" (1965, p. 101). Therefore, "The transformation in K must be replaced by the transformation in O, and K must be replaced by F [faith]" (Bion, 1970, p. 46); "the blast of an experience of this kind when you are actually there, when you are really exposed to it. It is, I can only say, 'indescribable'" (2013, p. 85).

But darkness was also a very concrete experience in Clari's nightmarish psychic reality. All the gripping horror situations occur when deep darkness descends upon her familiar world, when the texture of her real, familiar, homey environment violently and abruptly collapses into something awful, unthinkable, without meaning and without mercy—something that cannot be stopped or resisted; into a complete loss of safety, confidence, protectiveness, and orientation; into near-death.

This nightmarish darkness in Clari's experiential reality is intertwined with the "uncanny"—*"Das Unheimliche"* (Freud, 1919)—*heimlich* that becomes *unheimlich*, [5] "the class of the frightening which leads back to what is known of old and long familiar"—a lived experience (*"Erlebnis"*) (p. 220). It is a dark uncanny here. Clari's dreams of horror always began in her familiar environment with the eruption and encroachment of darkness: the repeated, dreadful, overwhelming "dreams of force" occurred in the real and familiar situation of her home and bedroom; the dream/memory-scene of the mortally battered baby is seen when she "got up to pee" there, in the dark; and the dream of total darkness and disorientation which immediately follows it occurs in her familiar neighborhood.

Is this striking shift from the familiar environment to darkness, void, and repetitive horror devoid of content, an expression of an awful, extremely traumatic rupture of unthinkable anxiety, of nameless dread? Or is it also a defensive reorganization of the traumatic, horrific experiences hidden in her familiar world?

These depths of the unknown, especially the most traumatic unknown, and "being totally in the dark" figuratively and concretely, both in Clari's experiential world and in the treatment experience, necessitate going beyond epistemological exploration to the ontological analytic work of being and becoming with-in the patient's experience, at-one-with the patient's innermost psychic reality—the unrepressed and unrepresented realm, level II, in the spectrum of analytic oneness that I have proposed, of the most unknown, unthinkable psychic reality; the deepest traumatic and non-communicating issues of human life.

It can also be said, following Freud's thinking in "The Uncanny" (1919), that I became the "double"—a human, alive, real, and present "double" in Clari's uncanniness,

> by mental processes leaping from one ... to another—by what we should call telepathy—so that the one possesses knowledge, feelings and experience in common with the other ... there is a doubling, dividing and interchanging of the self.
>
> (p. 234)

Botella and Botella (2005) expand on the idea of the analyst's "functioning or working as a double", which goes beyond "already known" countertransference meaning and thus gives access to the patient's unrepresentable areas that would otherwise remain traumatically unknown and unreachable (pp. 82–83).

Perhaps in order to enter and become-there, within Clari's impervious, inaccessible, yet needy inner world, I had to be in an unprotected, vulnerable, even paralyzed psychic state, to match the quality of her own core vulnerability. It is an intricate match; its essence, significance, and compatibility should be such that the analyst's/therapist's interconnected presence—like a transplant or chimeric antibodies in medicine—is not identified as a foreign body by the psyche's defense system and is therefore not attacked and rejected by it, but is able to become a new, living possibility. I would also add here Ogden's words:

> Being understood is terrifying [if] the person who understands is an other, an entirely separate person who lives outside of one's control, and at the same time knows one to the core and could, if he chose, cut one to the quick.
>
> (2016, p. 10)

It seems to me that the massive traumatic *realness* of early breakdown and madness (Winnicott, 1974, 1965), of "psychological disaster", "primitive catastrophe", and "the ruins of the psyche" (Bion, 1958, 1970), and of the uncanny (Freud, 1919) led them all to more radical ontological forms of psychoanalytic work and transformations in oneness: in Freud—the double, "for the 'double' was originally an insurance against the destruction of the ego, an 'energetic denial of the power of death'" (Freud, 1919, p. 235); in Winnicott's and Bion's late writings, despite the differences in their language, to their emphasis on the necessity for fundamental *being and experiencing* prior to understanding in the analytic work, and to "transformations in O" (Vermote,

2013). To my way of thinking, this traumatic realness also leads us from projective identification (of unbearable fear or phantasy) to what might be called *"projective realization"*[6] or *"projective embodiment"* *of catastrophic psychic realities that have already happened.* This is profoundly related to late Bion's groundbreaking words on the analyst's "being" and "becoming" the patient's innermost psychic reality-O that is unknown and unknowable, which enable reaching the deepest form of psychoanalytic (ontological) understanding:

> The psycho-analytic vertex is O. With this the analyst cannot be identified: he must *be* it. ... In so far as the analyst becomes O, he is able to know the events that are the *evolutions* of O. Restating this in terms of psycho-analytic experience, the psycho-analyst can know what the patient says, does, and appears to be, but cannot know the O of which the patient is an evolution: he can only "be" it.
>
> (1970, p. 27, italics in original)

With this in mind, let us return to Clari's treatment. In Clari's psychic reality, the traumatic, terrifying early experiences were massively dissociated, their contents warded off. She was caught within a persistent, gripping nightmarish scene of raw horror, with repeated, uncanny scenarios of utter darkness, loneliness, and desperation, while being in the grip of an overwhelming, inescapable anti-life force. She was crushed and stifled nearly to death, emotionally and somatically, depending for existence itself on a whim—a scene of total helplessness, of dissociated, unspeakable abuse and longing, and mere physical survival. There was also the retraumatization with which Clari came to me for treatment because of her former therapist's departure.

As the treatment evolved, Clari increasingly projected-forced these fundamental, central elements of her psychic reality into me—the coercive extreme dissociation of self-experience; the cognitive-affective paralysis with the gap in continuity of experience (Lichtenberg et al., 1992); the absence. Now, the experience of being inside a massive dissociative, blank process was occurring in *me—a vicarious self-state dissociation,* thus detaching and distancing it from her while she observed from without. But when I let it affect me, allowing it to be and become me, without understanding it but also without dread, carrying in me the knowledge from experience of having been repeatedly dissociated and absent—yet staying there, in the treatment, surviving, trying to hold and think the experience—it gradually became a therapeutic experience. The dissociation very slowly became a new kind of dissociation—*an attenuated, deferred dissociation,* because the dissociation in me—or, more precisely, in the interconnected entity of her-and-me—was no longer the extremely lonely, unmediated, life-defending dissociative self-experience of her, but a dissociative experience that was held differently within me, and within a human process—a massive yet sustained and tolerable one.

I quoted earlier Bion's words

If the analyst can take certain steps that enable him to 'see' what the patient sees, it is reasonable to suppose that the patient has likewise 'taken steps', though not necessarily the same ones, to enable him to 'see' what he sees.

(1970, p. 40)

Indeed, after months of my unchanging recurring sleep in Clari's treatment,

one session, while still in this deep sleep, I saw a kind of schematic drawing of a bright tunnel with a small black dot moving up and down in its center. This was the first time that I saw or felt something while in this state, and I awoke with an unfamiliar sense of relief.

And although I was unable to put it into words for me or for her, Clari came to the next session and told me the horrible dream/memory-scene of the mortally battered baby.

Thus, the externalization of the dissociation within and through me, and being within psyche-with-psyche connectedness, enabled Clari to dare approach, observe, and experience the dread of her inner self-other experiences. She could begin to dream, think, imagine, to risk exploring the traumatic contents of her massive uncanniness, which, until now, had been unknowable, unthinkable, extremely dissociated, and inaccessible, threatening her with desperation, collapse, madness, and dying. Fact-finding became self-finding. In this way, we went through and beyond the dissociation.

Finally, still along this line of deep patient-analyst interconnectedness, but looking at my "sleep" from a very different perspective—my sleep during Clari's treatment could be regarded as regression in the countertransference to a "good sleep" (suggested by Bollas, 1997, personal communication). When I actualized the capacity to fall asleep for Clari, she, too, was able to let herself fall soundly asleep (as in the dream of her falling asleep, in spite of the dark, in face-to-face togetherness with me). She could hold the hand of the terrified, lost little girl within herself and put her to bed, as in the first good dream that she dreamt, and begin to actualize "dream-space" (Khan, 1972) and inner space for remembering, which she was robbed of by her traumatic childhood. This is a "good sleep" that is created with and through another person. This point resonates with Ferenczi's (1932) early words: "a sleeping person is defenseless: When one is asleep, one relies on the safety of the house and the environment, otherwise one could not fall asleep" (p. 45).

Perhaps, at the end of all the explanations and beyond all explanations, I would dare to say that in this treatment, without knowing it at the time, amid the depths of not understanding and not knowing, there came into being an "*act of faith*" (Bion, 1970) and "area of faith" (Eigen, 1981)—out of my fundamental, profound belief and trust in the psychoanalytic process, in the deep connectedness of patient-and-analyst, in myself as an analyst; and not less important—out of Clari's persistence in treatment which grew into a great determination to intensify it, despite the dread that was strongly expressed in her dream just prior to the transition to analysis, as she opened the door to the unknown. It was an "act of faith" that came into being within the evolving oneness of me-and-Clari, Clari-and-me.

Afterword

In this account, I have restricted myself to what I experienced, came to understand, and did not understand about my "sleeping"—during the course of Clari's psychotherapy and shortly afterwards, at the beginning of the analysis. I chose not to use material from later in the analysis because I wanted to convey the quality of the experience for me at the time—its grip, its experiential vicissitudes, its unknowns and unfoldings. Yet, I would like to add that during the analysis, I no longer experienced "sleeping". It seems that this was a phase in the treatment that Clari and I had already lived through. *T(w) ogether.*

Notes

1 In modern physics, different paradigms of classical physics and quantum mechanics co-exist. Whereas classical physics (and classical psychoanalysis) are based on assumptions of linear causality, determinism, and a sharp separation between observer and observed, quantum physics introduced into scientific thinking essential principles of uncertainty and inseparability of observer and observed, the crucial formative effect of the process of observation, and the fundamental organization of unbroken wholeness that underlies our perceived world of separateness at the fundamental particle level (Eshel, 2017a, 2019a).
2 Bion, 1965, p. 15. According to Neville Symington (2016), it is called O by Bion, for "Ontology". Winnicott (probably in 1968) joins these two words by writing about "ontological origin" (p. 213).
3 "Be at one with" (Bion, 1967, 1970); "become 'at-one' with the patient's experience" (Bion, 1995, pp. 96, 107); "Being-at-one-with" (Winnicott, 1971, p. 94; Ogden, 2015, p. 294).
4 Regarding this dream, I encountered an article in *The New York Times* that described phenomena such as a sensed presence, terror, strong immobility, a crushing pressure, and struggle for breath as the mysterious "sleep paralysis" (Kristof, 1999).
5 When I asked a native German speaker to explain the word *unheimlich*, she said, "It is a child in darkness, a lurking danger."
6 Also used by Wassermann (personal communication, 2021) but in a somewhat different sense.

References

Bergstein, A. (2014). Beyond the spectrum: Fear of breakdown, catastrophic change and the unrepressed unconscious. *Rivista Di Psicoanalisi*, 60, 847–868.

Bion, F. (1995/2014). The days of our years. In C. Mawson (Ed.), *The complete works of W. R. Bion* (Vol. XV, pp. 91–111). Karnac.

Bion, W.R. (1958). On arrogance. In: *Second thoughts* (pp. 86–92). Maresfield Library/Karnac.

Bion, W.R. (1962). *Learning from experience.* Maresfield Library/Karnac.

Bion, W.R. (1965). *Transformations.* Maresfield Library/Karnac.

Bion, W.R. (1967). Notes on memory and desire. *The Psychoanalytic Forum, 2,* 272–273.

Bion, W.R. (1970). *Attention and interpretation.* Maresfield Library/Karnac.

Bion, W.R. (1992). *Cogitations.* Karnac.

Bion, W.R. (2005). *The Italian seminars.* Karnac.

Bion, W.R. (2013). *Los Angeles seminars and supervisions,* Ed. J. Aguayo & B. Malin. Karnac.

Bohm, D. (1980). *Wholeness and the implicate order.* Routledge/Kegan Paul.

Botella, C., & Botella, S. (2005). *The work of psychic figurability: Mental states without representation.* Brunner-Routledge/The New Library of Psychoanalysis.

Eigen, M. (1981). The area of faith in Winnicott, Lacan, and Bion. *Int. J. Psychoanal.,* 62, 413–433.

Eshel, O. (1998). "Black holes," deadness and existing analytically. *Int. J. Psychoanal.,* 79, 1115–1130.

Eshel, O. (2001). Whose sleep is it, anyway? Or "night moves". *Int. J. Psychoanal.,* 82, 545–562.

Eshel, O. (2004). Let it be and become me: Notes on containing, identification, and the possibility of being. *Contemp. Psychoanal.,* 40, 323–351.

Eshel, O. (2017a). From extension to revolutionary change in clinical psychoanalysis: The radical influence of Bion and Winnicott. *Psychoanalytic Quarterly,* 86(4), 753–794.

Eshel, O. (2017b). Into the depths of a "black hole" and deadness. In A. Reiner (Ed.), *Of things invisible to mortal sight: Celebrating the work of James S. Grotstein* (pp. 39–68). Karnac.

Eshel, O. (2019a). *The emergence of analytic oneness: Into the heart of psychoanalysis.* Routledge.

Eshel, O. (2019b). The vanished last scream: Winnicott and Bion. *Psychoanalytic Quarterly,* 88(1), 111–140.

Eshel, O., & Zeligman, Z. (2017). *Was it or was it not? When shadows of sexual abuse emerge in psychoanalytic treatment.* Carmel.

Ferenczi, S. (1932). 24 February 1932: Trauma in an unconscious state. In J. Dupont (Ed.), Trans. M. Balint & N.Z. Jackson (1988), *The clinical diary of Sandor Ferenczi* (pp. 45–32). Harvard Univ. Press.

Freud, S. (1900). The interpretation of dreams (part 2). In *S.E.* (Vol. 5).

Freud, S. (1915). The unconscious. In *S.E.* (Vol. 14, pp. 161–215).

Freud, S. (1919). The 'uncanny'. In *S.E.* (Vol. 17).

Freud, S. (1923). The ego and the id. In *S.E.* (Vol. 19, pp. 31–66).

Gribbin, J. (1992). *In search of the edge of time: Black holes, white holes, wormholes.* Penguin Books.

Hawking, S. (1988). *A brief history of time: From the big bang to black holes.* Bantam Books.

Hawking, S. (1993). *Black holes and baby universes, and other essays.* Bantam.

Khan, M.M. (1972). The use and abuse of dream in psychic experience. In *The privacy of the self* (1974, pp. 306–315). Hogarth.

Kristof, N.D. (1999). Alien abduction? Science calls it sleep paralysis. *New York Times*, 7 July 1999.

Levine, H.B. (2022). *Affect, representation and language: Between the silence and the cry*, Routledge.

Levine, H., Reed, G.S., & Scarfone, D. (Eds.) (2013). *Unrepresented states and the construction of meaning: Clinical and theoretical contribution*. Karnac.

Lichtenberg, J.D., et al. (1992). *Self and motivational systems: Toward a theory of psychoanalytic technique*. Analytic Press.

Ogden, T.H. (2001). Reading Winnicott. In *Conversations at the frontier of dreaming* (pp. 203–235). Karnac.

Ogden, T.H. (2015). Intuiting the truth of what's happening: On Bion's "Notes on memory and desire". *Psychoanalytic Quarterly*, 84, 285–306.

Ogden, T.H. (2016). *Reclaiming unlived life*. Routledge.

Ogden, T.H. (2019). Ontological psychoanalysis or "what do you want to be when you grow up?" *Psychoanalytic Quarterly*, 88(4), 661–684.

Rodman, R.F. (Ed.) (1987). *The spontaneous gesture: Selected letters of D.W. Winnicott*. Harvard University Press.

Symington, N. (2016). Group seminar, Tel Aviv University, Tel Aviv.

Vermote, R. (2013). *The undifferentiated zone of psychic functioning: An integrative approach and clinical implications*. Presentation at the European Psychoanalytical Federation (EPF) Conference, Basel, March 24. See also: Vermote, R. (2013). The undifferentiated zone of psychic functioning. European Psychoanalytical Federation, *Psychoanalysis in Europe Bulletin*, 67, 16–27.

Winnicott, D.W. (1945). Primitive emotional development. In *Through paediatrics to psychoanalysis* (1992, pp. 145–156). Karnac.

Winnicott, D.W. (1963). Communicating and not communicating leading to a study of certain opposites. In *The maturational processes and the facilitating environment* (1979, pp. 179–192). Hogarth Press.

Winnicott, D.W. (1965). The psychology of madness: A contribution from *explorations* psychoanalysis. In C. Winnicott, R. Shepherd, & M. Davis (Eds.) (1989), *Psychoanalytic* (pp. 119–129). Karnac.

Winnicott, D.W. (1968). Thinking and symbol-formation. In C. Winnicott, R. Shepherd, & M. Davis (Eds.), *Psycho-analytic explorations* (1989, pp. 213–216). Karnac Books.

Winnicott, D.W. (1971). *Playing and reality*. Penguin.

Winnicott, D.W. (1974). Fear of breakdown. *International Review of Psycho-Analysis*, 1, 103–107.

Chapter 7

A personal perspective on the somato-psychic realm based on Bion's contributions

João Carlos Braga

Psychoanalysis is a living body of knowledge that is constantly expanding with contributions from those who practice it. Basic psychoanalytic concepts—even the most basic ones—are frequently modifying, fulfilling the objectives of psychoanalysis, i.e., the scientific study of the psyche. The concept of the somato-psychic realm illustrates this fundamental condition. This concept emerges as a new realm from the prior development of the primordial mind by W.R. Bion, which in turn emerged from the seminal concept of the unconscious by Freud.

Based on ideas by Freud and Melanie Klein and on his own experience, Bion developed an approach to psychoanalytic theory and practice that has shifted our view of the mind from one that starts on a biological level (*instincts*) to another that starts on a psychological level (*thinking* and *being*). Bion's approach has opened new scientific frontiers to the psychoanalytic comprehension of mental functioning. Due to the heuristic and hermeneutic qualities of his approach, Bion's legacy has the peculiar characteristic of something not to be learned and owned but conquered and integrated into each analyst's mind based on their own experiences. These characteristics make the study of Bion's ideas a never-ending task that unfolds with the important bias of being developed from a *personal perspective*.

Bion and the somato-psychic realm—a historic background

Many of Bion's insights are so novel that they still startle 40 years after they were published. The idea of a primordial mind is one of Bion's keen insights still waiting to be developed; the somato-psychic realm is part of the concept of the primordial mind.

The somato-psychic realm belongs to Bion's conjectures that the mind has a bedrock—a proto-mental personality—modeled after a prenatal mind that functions independently from the development of postnatal experiences. Bion tentatively named this form of psychic functioning *primordial*. In his words: "that is what seems to me to be one of the fundamental discoveries of

DOI: 10.4324/9781003534365-7

psychoanalysis: archaic states of mind, archaic thoughts and ideas, primitive patterns of behaviour are all detectable in the most civilized, cultivated people" (Bion, 1977, p. 38).

Bion's statement that manifestations of this archaic heritage "crops up very frequently in many different analyses" (Bion, 1978, Supervision A5) conveys the impression that, among his ideas, this is probably the one that has received the least attention and has been least integrated into the mainstream of psychoanalytic thinking. Another way to look at this would be to say that Bion's thinking regarding the primordial mind is still far ahead of our current psychoanalytic thinking ability.

Bion died before elaborating his contributions on the primordial mind to a more satisfactory level. Had he enjoyed a few more years of a psycho-analytically productive life, we could have today a psychoanalytic model of mental functioning in which the most elemental aspects of the mind would have a more important role than the one currently recognized. With his death, the conceptual tools that he was developing lost the only person who knew how to work them. Several years passed before psychoanalysts started unearthing this scientific treasure, accepting its importance, and creating a medium capable of further expanding his original thoughts.

In Bion's communications, the primordial mind appears as inaccessible to being known, directly experienced, or observable. Bion referred to the primordial mind as imaginative, the product of rational conjectures that "may take years to confirm scientifically" (Bion & Bion, 1981, p. 83). Intentionally, he did not entirely organize his ideas, as he was probably fully aware that they required further investigation and confirmation by other psychoanalysts.

Four decades after Bion published his ideas on the primordial mind, psy-choanalysts still struggle to identify the presence of this *primordial personality* that evolves amalgamated with the postnatal personality, and to find ways to deal with the primordial mind in their practices. For this task, they rely on Bion's insights and their own clinical experiences. To examine the concept of the primordial mind, we must first give it a more comprehensive look before delving into its particularities. One hypothesis to consider at this point is that Bion, at that time, had a hunch that he was glimpsing a *quantum psycho-analysis* that was quite different from a psychoanalysis capable of being organized in knowable deterministic concepts. The problem of finding a sci-entific model for psychoanalysis still haunts us, and the quantum theory as a model seems increasingly helpful for this purpose. As an example of the pre-sence of this idea in Bion's mind, we find the following passage at the end of *Caesura,* where he presents his version of Freud's words: "there is much more continuity between anatomically appropriate *quanta* and the *waves* of con-scious thought and feeling than the impressive caesura of transference and countertransference would have us believe" (Bion, 1975 [1977], p. 57; my italics).

The somato-psychic realm

Let us consider two major reasons to study the somato-psychic realm, singling it out from its cradle, the primordial mind. The first is Bion's continuous striving to approach the Origin (O) of the mind, and the second is his interest in discriminating two different psychosomatic phenomena, one with a starting point in the body (*somato-psychotic*, as named by Bion) and the other with a starting point in the mind (*psycho-somatic*). Both movements have been treated as part of the concepts of psychosomatic and primordial mind.

Bion identified the somato-psychic realm in the following passage:

> ... unconscious and which may even be pre-natal, or pre-birth of a psyche or a mental life, but is part of a physical life in which at some stage a physical impulse is immediately translated into a physical action. ... Can we detect in these expressions of conscious rational communications vestiges of something coming from a part of the personality which is in fact physical?
>
> (Bion, 1975 [1977], p. 55)

The somato-psychic realm is constituted by "primordial ideas and feelings which have never been conscious" (Bion, 1980, pp. 20–21), and their seal is "the kind of fear one would have if no check on it at all was produced by the higher levels of the mind" (Bion, 1976, p. 319). In this last passage, Bion referred to *fear* as representing the group of primordial feelings; in other moments, he tentatively referred to it as *sub-thalamic fear* (Bion, 1976, p. 319) and *nameless dread* (Bion, 1962a, p. 116).

Bion's proposal of the existence of the primordial mind directs our attention to the challenges that mind and body must face to *talk* to each other and *make arrangements* to reach an improbable peaceful outcome. This approach calls attention to two different dimensions—one that is possible to know as facts (i.e., mind and body) and the other as models (i.e., Psyche-Soma and Soma-Psyche, see below)—tentatively personifying the ineffable reality of mind and body. Bion's play with words offers us a savory approach to this issue:

MIND: Hullo! Where have you sprung from?
BODY: What—you again? I am Body; you can call me Soma if you like. Who are you?
MIND: Call me Psyche—Psyche-Soma.
BODY: Soma-Psyche
MIND: We must be related.
BODY: Never—not if I can help it.
MIND: Oh, come. Not as bad as that is it?

BODY: Worse. You got us into this air. Luckily I brought some liquid with me. What are you doing?(Bion, 1979, p. 4–5)

André Green (1998) made two fundamental observations on this issue. The first indicating that "thinking is often confused with psychic activity" (p. 651) and the second discriminating between "psychic events rooted in the body", "thoughts without a thinker", and "thinking":

> The conclusion is that we have to distinguish between *psychic events*, which have to be understood as rooted in the body, *thoughts without a thinker*, which are very close to this primitive psychic activity and *thinking, which has to be thought by a thinker* and therefore can be communicated to another thinker. Bion's hypothesis that emotional experience is the matrix of the mind is related to the closeness of the thoughts without a thinker with the models drawn from bodily activity. Thinking is a digestion of the mind.
>
> (Green, 1998, p. 652, italics in original)

According to this approach, "*psychic events, which have to be understood as rooted in the body*" would refer to the primordial mind. It would encompass what Bion conjecturally described as phylogenetic endeavor plus prenatal records and postnatal experiences that have their starting point in the thalamic-adrenal-gonadal axis. These somato-psychic elements would appear amalgamated or infiltrated in elements of the developed mind.

Of note, Green's formulations do not overlap with Bion's ideas on the primordial mind. Green's references to the primordial mind convey the idea of precursors of experiences that are part of Bion's theory of thinking, while Bion's ideas refer to a prenatal personality.

We can consider Bion's ideas as supported in physical experiences of the caesura between the prenatal and the postnatal life and with the presence of non-myelinated neurons in the fetus and their myelinization after birth. For the fetus, the imprint of the operational nervous system would be not in the brain cortex but on more primordial structures (thalamus, adrenals, gonads).

The somato-psychic realm and the primordial mind: Establishing a framework for discussion

We have no sensuous evidence of the primordial mind or representations of physical experiences that show its existence; we can only think about it and represent the elements that we acknowledge as its manifestations. In Bion's words, "the mental counterpart with the inward eye" (Bion, 1965, p. 102).

Sandler (2005, p. 468) offers a fundamental alert on these matters:

If it is ineffable, the task of formulating it verbally is doomed to failure. The relative success of the formulations depends on the listener's experience, and intuition concerning the apprehension of the Platonic-Kantian numinous realm, the unconscious itself.

Bion privileged the study of these primordial manifestations during his last three years of life (1976–1979). His ideas are scattered across different communications, including his last publications[1], seminars across different countries,[2] and dozens of recorded supervisions that he held during a visit to Brazil in 1978.[3] These communications show his effort to identify and point out the importance of working psychoanalytically with these remains of the primordial personality that emerge amalgamated with more developed layers of the personality.

Bion considered the primordial mind to be part of a negative dimension of the mind, i.e., as having a non-sensuous existence. In his words,

I am suggesting that besides the conscious and unconscious states of mind, there can be another one. The nearest I can get to giving it a provisional title is the inaccessible state of mind. It can become inaccessible because the foetus gets rid of it as soon as it can.

(Bion, 1977, p. 50)

From the manifestations that we conjecture as being somato-psychic, we must consider two possibilities. One is that these manifestations are remains of a prenatal personality, an idea postulated explicitly by Bion, and the other is that they are raw materials from postnatal experiences that have not undergone the psychic processes that allow a sensuous or emotional experience to evolve to a thought generated by the thinker. Bion only briefly mentioned this second possibility, which was later expanded by Green (1998, p. 652). To address this concept in the clinical setting, Bion recurred to the idea of wild thoughts, a kind of thought without a thinker (Bion, 1977, p. 27), thoughts in potentia but never born to the mind, i.e., pre-conceptions waiting for realizations. Their realm would follow the rules of the autonomic nervous system and hypothalamic-adrenal-gonadal axis, structures developed before birth.

Regarding the prenatal personality, Bion conjectured that the fetus has sensuous (visual and auditory) experiences, proto-feelings, and proto-ideas (Bion, 1975 [1977], p. 44; 1976, p. 318), and a primordial form of projective identification (Bion, 1976, p. 318) that tries to expel these painful stimuli.

Bion introduced these ideas of a primordial mind in *Caesura* (1975 [1977], p. 44):

Events sometimes take place in the consulting room, where there are present only myself and a grown man or woman, which suggest feelings that I could describe as envy, love, hate, sex, but which seem to have an intense and unformed character. It's convenient to fall back on physiology and anatomy to borrow ideas in order to express my feelings about some of these events; to think of some of the feelings which the patient is expressing as being sub-thalamic, or sympathetic, or para-sympathetic.

When we approach Bion's investigations of the primordial mind, we identify references to models, conjectures, conceptions, and even concepts, but we find no hypotheses or theories, i.e., a kind of a phylogenetic-ontogenetic perspective. For example, when Bion points out that the experiences of being all alone and dependent, of the urge to exist, and of a primitive conscience are structures of the primordial mind, we can conjecture the hidden presence of the ancestors of the ego, the id, and the superego, respectively.

The primordial mind and the somato-psychic realm: Furthering a few points

Based on various supervisions that Bion held in São Paulo in 1978, we know that, during that period, he was essentially working with the principle that the analyst must intuit "the date of the quality he is observing" (Bion & Bion, 1981, p. 25). This same observation is possible in the description by José Américo Junqueira de Mattos (2016) regarding his own analysis with Bion during that very same period. In Bion's remarks in both situations—supervisions and Junqueira's analysis—he was basing his intervention on his own intuitions. Bion's observations called attention sometimes to the operative presence of the knowing and not knowing processes or to the dimension of becoming reality, and at other times to that of the primordial mind. At rare moments, his observations focused on the functioning of the symbolic mind described by Freud or on the primitive mind described by Melanie Klein. He was evidently working with the model of a multidimensional mind. In the clinic, the analyst's intuitive grasp of the stage of development of that which is undergoing transformation offers data for adjusting his or her approach to the evolving emotional experience carrying a fragment of psychic reality.

Like Freud's efforts to create a scientific approach to mental life, Bion turned his focus to the Origin of the mind in the interaction between body and psyche functioning. He focused on two patterns involving the encounter of both the dimensions, i.e., the psychosomatic and the somato-psychic, indicating that pressures to discharge stimuli can originate in the body or the mind, with the manifestation appearing in the other dimension. A frequent analogy that Bion used was that of the two faces of the hand, which can be observed as existing separately but are parts of the same hand. In *Evidence* (1976, p. 318) and *Caesura* (1975 [1977], p. 51), Bion resorted to more sophisticated analogies, those of Picasso's painting on glass, which can be seen from two different angles, and of a mountain that can be seen differently from various cardinal points.

Bion's use of two notations—somato-psychotic and somato-psychic—also requires some clarification. Personally, I have found no records of Bion discussing these different notations and wonder whether we could look at them as discriminations between the psychotic phenomena and the phenomena proper to the primordial mind. The latter are not psychotic phenomena, as Bion recognized them only after developing the concept of thoughts without a thinker, taking as a model the prenatal personality. Would somato-psychic refer to a natural condition present in all of us, in which somatic needs drive the individual to psychological needs, as in hunger and sexual impulses? Would somato-psychotic be a notation for a somatic stimulus that turns into an emotional impulse that achieves a distorted representation? The practicing analyst has a privileged condition to investigate both conditions:

> In the relationship I have been describing—pre-natal<–>post-natal—the individual often behaves as if his wisdom and intelligence would be contaminated if he allowed himself to recognize that his body thought; conversely, that his physique would suffer if he allowed his body to know what his mind thought.

> (Bion, 1979, pp. 128–129)

Somato-psychic realm: Bodily structures and sensorial and emotional experiences providing elements for a potential matching between container and contained

With his theory of knowledge (1962b, 1963, 1965), Bion created conceptual tools that allow us to think about the mysterious process in which an emotion or a sensorial experience is transformed (or not) into mental tissue. But how about proprioceptive stimuli? How should we think about stimuli that originate in the internal organs and can—or cannot—reach the brain through the autonomic nervous system, or vice-versa? For example, when a person blushes, is it the emotion that appears as a somatic manifestation, or is it a somatic manifestation that appears as an emotion to the mind? Or are these two different faces of a single process? Freud and Bion cautiously treated this area with mystery and awe.

While attempting to think about the somato-psychic realm, we can follow Freud and Bion and "fly into fantasy" (Bion, 1976, p. 318) with the help of Green. The *psychic events rooted in the body* (Green, 1998, p. 652) can be seen as the primitive psychic activity undifferentiated from its somatic base (Freud), the beta elements in Bion's theory:

> The main difference between Bion and Freud could be that for Freud the drives always had their source in the most inner part of the body, whereas for Bion, β-elements may also arise from external stimuli in the primordial mind.

> (Green, 1998, p. 653)

Resorting to Bion's theory of thinking, we can build more bridges to overcome the caesura between body and psyche. We can take the development of the process of creating a thought by the thinker as a necessary sequence in four stages, which can be identified in the first twelve chapters of *Learning from Experience* (Bion, 1962b). The very first step would be the mating of elements functioning as potential "containers" and "contained". The emotional experience (Love, Hatred, Knowledge) occurring with the achievement of a container/contained relationship would be the second step, the very beginning of the thought-producing process. We could wonder whether this would be the leap from soma to psychic activity and its decisive step. Perhaps only a small part of the successful mating of container/contained and the emotional experiences so generated will be linked to the activity of consciousness. If this step is not fulfilled, these proto-thoughts ("psychic events rooted in the body") remain as *thoughts without a thinker*: soma and psyche remaining indistinguishable as parts of an undifferentiated operative unconscious. If consciousness is added to the emotional experience, the necessary conditions to proceed to an alpha-function operation are complete and an alpha-element is generated; thus, oneiric thoughts are formed and thinking quality is acquired.

Green's differentiation between no-thoughts ("psychic events rooted in the body"), potential thinking ("thoughts without a thinker"), and abstract thinking ("thoughts" produced by a thinker) is a remarkable conception. Based on this conception, the primordial mind would be constituted by elements of raw and crude nature and, thus, not workable as thoughts for the thinker. They would have to be expelled from the psyche through the action of a primitive apparatus prior to the thinking one, the projective identification apparatus (Bion, 1962a, p. 117).

The somato-psychic primordial functioning and the theory of transformations

We examined until this point the primordial functioning of the somato-psychic realm from the perspective of the theory of knowledge (Bion, 1962a, 1962b, 1963, 1965). What happens when we look at the primordial mind after the theory of transformations (Bion, 1965)?

The theory of transformations can be seen as a turning point in Bion's ideas, his attempt in 1965 to encompass all the different psychoanalytic transformations recognizable in clinical practice. It offered instruments for him to expand the psychoanalytic domains beyond the knowing/not-knowing dimensions. Based on this theory, we think about the mind as composed of a set of different dimensions. Psychic manifestations of primordial experiences, like the somato-psychic realm, can be examined side by side with other dimensions of mental experiences, i.e., reason, knowing (K), not knowing (-K), hallucinosis, and being or becoming reality. Bion did not seek to include the manifestations of the primordial mind into his theory of transformations. In fact, he presented his ideas on the primordial mind one decade after he had presented the theory of transformations.

The integration of the primordial mind into the theory of transformations was a contribution by Celia F. Korbivcher, with her proposals of the autistic transformations (2002) and non-integrated transformations (2013). Autistic transformations are characterized by transformations occurring in an autistic medium in the absence of the notion of internal and external objects. Clinically, they appear as auto-sensuous activity, lack of emotional life, and an experience of emptiness by the analyst. The relationship between *me* and *not me* is mediated by sensation objects—autistic shapes and autistic objects, as described by F. Tustin. Regarding the non-integrated transformations, they received this name because they occur in a primordial medium, that is, a medium not integrated with the developed mind. They are characterized by manifestations without a psychic representation, states of extreme vulnerability expressed by the dread of falling into a black hole, of spilling and dissolving, and an intense fear of losing the notion of one's own existence.

Transformations of the primordial mind are far more difficult to follow than the other forms of psychoanalytic transformations since they only become accessible through infiltrations in the developed parts of the personality. As these are non-sensuous psychoanalytic objects, we must identify the presence of mindless manifestations. The challenge to the analyst is to discern what can be conjectured as "embryonic" remains and, on the other hand, the experience of object relationships.

Somato-psychic manifestations

Somato-psychic manifestations come to light as bodily symptoms, varieties of acting out, or rational communications. In the last case, the manifestations look like thoughts, but only resemble thinking activity; in fact, they are powerful emotions hidden by rationalizations.

When manifestations of the primordial mind are at stake, a common general observation for the analyst is a lack of emotional, oneiric, and cognitive fluency in the analytic relationship. The analysand repeats the same themes over and over again, with little changes. He or she has an emotional tone indicating great involvement with actual problems, while carefully avoiding any approach to the inner life and emotional experiences emerging in the analytic relationship. Transference is far from being a significant issue.

In the session, analyst and analysand depart from very different points of origin to create their representations of the experiences that they are living. The analyst is expected to identify that they are not sharing the same emotional experience. The analysand's manifestation is distant from the experience of the session and is lived as something strange. The analyst faces an area where alpha function has not worked. The analytic investigation reveals that the analysand is aware of his or her pain but does not live this pain as suffering. The manifestations are out of reach to interpretations based on classic psychoanalytic theories, such as Freud's and Klein's understanding of the mind, as well as of Bion's theory of thinking.

The analyst living this type of analytic experience has feelings of emptiness. The analysand pressures the analyst with not-so-subtle pleas for reassurance and expects explanations. Instead of feelings or emotions, the analyst finds rationalizations, forms of acting out, or physical manifestations depending on the autonomic nervous system.

A closer examination of the analysand's communications allows access to experiences of intense terror and guilt, both feelings being powerfully and dreadfully experienced. These feelings frequently infiltrate rationalized expressions that resemble thinking formed from real experiences, and such infiltrations create confusion with real fear, phobia, or persecutory terror. Fear originating from the somato-psychic realm as its hallmark the mind/soma incongruency.

Mental areas of arrested emotional development are frequently spotted in an analysis. In the absence of manifest change after analytic work, the analyst should consider the presence of infiltrations of a somato-psychic condition in the clinical material. Although present since the beginning of the analysis, somato-psychic manifestations often become more clearly accessible to analytic work only after deep elaboration of the functioning layers of the differentiated mind.

Observations from some long-term analyses (those lasting more than ten years, for example) reveal that manifestations of the somato-psychic realm become more integrated into the analysand's mental functioning but never disappear. The analysand's entire personality develops more tolerance of these manifestations and deals more confidently with them. This develops as part of the analysand's increased contact with the different dimensions of their mental life. Within the scope of this chapter, we could say that *Psyche-Soma* and *Soma-Psyche,* in the dialogue reproduced above (Bion, 1979, pp. 4–5), would then have the potential to reach a more harmonious outcome. Analysands achieve a condition of better acceptance of their limits and possibilities, although the mind/body relationship maintains areas of strain but with diminished violence. Terror and baseless guilt do not disappear but are mitigated by enchantment with the possibilities of personality expansion, increased autonomy in personal life, and the analysand's sense of increased responsibility for themselves and their relationships. These analysands show a strong attachment to the analytic process and an interest in increasingly deepening their experiences. Their analyses often tend to be endless; decades can pass. The analytic process is recognized as valuable and rewarding. The more involved the analysands become with their mental lives, the more easily they recognize and appreciate the reality of their own existence and its somato-psychic dimension (Rezze & Braga, 2019). In short, they show increased satisfaction with the way they live their lives.

The somato-psychic realm, Bion, and the practicing psychoanalyst

When addressing analytical experiences, Bion always displayed a cautious attitude and frequently used interrogative sentences. He was perhaps fully aware that the object of his studies was impossible to be determined and that it could only be considered as probable. His reference to "quanta" and "waves" suggests that he was thinking with quantum physics as his model and that he was aware of the meaning of this perspective for analytic practice: "this involves taking a different view about the obstacles to psychoanalytic progress, the development of the relationship between analyst and analysand, and considering phenomena which present themselves in the actual analytic situation" (Bion, 1975 [1977], p. 56).

In his writings during this period we find several references to the way that Bion clinically approached the primordial mind. Notably, he displayed a general view of a multidimensional mind, but during those three years he did so with stronger emphasis on the analyst intervening based on the inner experience of the analysand. Below are some examples highlighting Bion's ideas on the management of somato-psychic manifestations:

In *Caesura* (1975 [1977], p. 55), Bion wrote: "can we detect in these expressions of conscious rational communications vestiges of something coming from a part of the personality which is in fact physical?" In *Evidence* (1976, p. 319), Bion clearly presents the analyst's challenges:

> Supposing we are in fact always dealing with some kind of psychoso-matic condition. Is it any good talking to a highly articulate person in highly articulate terms? Is it possible that, if feelings of intense fear, self-hatred, can seep up into a state of mind in which they can be translated into action, the reverse is true? Is it possible to talk to the soma in such a way that the psychosis is able to understand, or vice versa?

In Supervisions A5 and A6 (Bion, São Paulo, 1978), Bion offers some hints of his way of clinically dealing with manifestations that he acknowledged as being from the primordial mind:

> I don't think I would want to say anything of that to her, at the moment, because I'm not sure whether the patient could stand it—I would prob-ably want to hear some more. But in the meantime, I would keep to myself the fact that this is a fundamental, basic guilt.
> ... Now the point about this: what should I say to the patient? What interpretation should I give? Or shall I remain silent? Now, if I remain

silent, then I am stepping into the position of being the conscience, which is no good to her; I need more information and, therefore, I'd prefer to remain silent until I heard some more. But if I were the analyst, I would not really know whether I could afford to wait, or whether it would make her more than ever, frightened of me as the unhelpful and hostile conscience.

Of course, the problem still exists [as?] to what the analyst would say to the patient, because whatever the analyst says to the patient, is an action; he's really doing something. I would have thought that the point that he needs to be aware of is the murderous quality of that conscience, which hates a happy and pleasurable and successful intercourse, verbal or otherwise. So, I think that it would be useful for him, to be aware of, so that he could make allowances for that kind of murderous moral standard, which would really mean the destruction of any creative activity.

And in *The Dawn of Oblivion* (1979, p. 129):

Psycho-analytic conjecture can be dismissed as too fanciful, but it is possible that a psycho-analyst might reconcile one of his analysands to respect what his body is trying to tell him and even persuade his body to have some respect for his mind.

Closing words

The somato-psychic realm may be seen as one of the frontiers in which psychoanalytic practice and theory push the limits of our access to the mind. The experiences and knowledge so far gathered about the somato-psychic realm have not been fully integrated into the mainstream of the psychoanalytic field.

We are now furthering Bion's initial evaluation that we are dealing with "imaginative conjectures". We are discussing more than ideas "which may take years to confirm scientifically" (Bion & Bion, 1981, p. 83). These words are a constant reminder about the way that psychoanalysis develops. We often start with "imaginative conjectures" in clinical practice, and the analysand requires time to reach the recognition that what he or she is experiencing are actually manifestations of psychic reality.

Notes

1 *Caesura* (1975 [1977]), *Evidence* (1976), *On a Quotation from Freud* (1976), *Emotional Turbulence* (1976), *Making the Best of a Bad Job* (1979), and the trilogy *A Memoir of the Future* (1975, 1977, 1979).
2 Los Angeles (1976), New York (1977), Rome (1977), London (Tavistock, 1976–1979), São Paulo (1978).
3 We owe this rich legacy to the dedicated work by Dr. José Américo Junqueira de Mattos, who collected the recorded supervisions, transcribed the dialogues in English into audio tapes, and translated them into Portuguese. Some of these

supervisions are being published with comments by Brazilian psychoanalysts. The first volume was published by Routledge in 2017, *Bion in Brazil*, edited by José Américo Junqueira de Mattos, Gisèle Mattos Brito, and Howard Levine.

References

Bion, W.R. (1962a). A theory of thinking. *Int. J. Psychoanal.*, 43.

Bion, W.R. (1962b). *Learning from experience*. W. Heinemann.

Bion, W.R. (1963). *Elements of psycho-analysis*. W. Heinemann.

Bion, W.R. (1965/1991). *Transformations*. Maresfield Library.

Bion, W.R. (1975 [1977]). Caesura. In *Two papers: The grid and caesura*. Imago Ed.

Bion, W.R. (1976). Evidence. In F. Bion (Ed.) (1994), *Clinical seminars and other works*. Karnac Books.

Bion, W.R. (1977/1997). *Taming wild thoughts*, Ed. F. Bion. Karnac Books.

Bion, W.R. (1978). Supervisions A5, A6, A35, S12. Audiotape of supervision given at Brazilian Psychoanalytic Society of São Paulo. Transcription and notation by J.A. Junqueira de Mattos.

Bion, W.R. (1979). *The dawn of oblivion*. Book 3 of *A memoir of the future*. Clunie Press.

Bion, W.R. (1980). *Bion in New York and São Paulo*. Clunie Press.

Bion, W.R., & Bion, F. (1981). *A key to "A memoir of the future"*. Clunie Press.

Green, A. (1998). The primordial mind and the work of the negative. *Int. J. Psych.*, 79, 649–685.

Junqueira de Mattos, J.A. (2016). Impressions of my analysis with Dr. Bion. In H. Levine & G. Civitarese (Eds.), *The W. R. Bion tradition lines of development; Evolution of theory and practice over the decade*. Karnac Books.

Korbivcher, C.F. (2002). The theory of transformations and autistic states. Autistic transformations: a proposal. In C.F. Korbivcher (2014), *Autistic transformations*. Karnac Books.

Korbivcher, C.F. (2013). Bion and the unintegrated phenomena: Falling, dissolving, and spilling. In H. Levine & D. Power (Eds.) (2016), *Engaging primitive anxieties of the emerging self. The legacy of Frances Tustin*. Karnac Books.

Rezze, C.J., & Braga, J.C. (2019). Authentic pleasure: Capture of moments of unison with reality. In A. Alisobhani & G. Corstorphine, *Explorations in Bion's "O"*. Routledge.

Sandler, P.C. (2005). *The language of Bion – A dictionary of concepts*. Karnac Books.

Chapter 8

The primordial mind and the body
The "no-body"[1] and being a body

Celia Fix Korbivcher

> Can any method of communication be sufficiently 'sharp' to cross that caesura toward postnatal conscious thought back to the prenatal, in which thoughts and ideas have their counterpart in 'times' or 'levels' where are they not thoughts or ideas?
>
> (Bion, 1977, p. 127)

As we know, some individuals reach adulthood without having developed an integrated self. What can also be observed is that these people go to enormous lengths to produce the appearance of what they suppose is socially expected of them, without having formed an interior world that occupies their bodies, an interior world capable of supporting these efforts and making them meaningful.

Many commit themselves to bodybuilding and other types of physical exercises, caring for their appearance, and mimicking the image of someone muscular and powerful, in short, mimicking a fully integrated person. The body, however, can often serve as armor, through which they seek protection when faced with the vulnerability they are exposed to in the presence of another, separate person.

They frequently complain that they feel uncomfortable in their own body, experiencing it as separate sprawled pieces that do not form a whole and isn't integrated with their mind. They operate most of the time in primordial mental states. For them, the awareness of separation from the object has not been fully established. The body is their main means of expression. They are especially attracted to bodily sensations they experience from contact with another, rather than the fantasies that might arise from such contact.

Some of our more challenging patients operate with mental states like those described above.

Pedro, 20 years old, mentions in one of his sessions:

> I was thinking about this week's series of exercises. I want to work on my strength ... I had a good upper body workout with my arms, but my leg

DOI: 10.4324/9781003534365-8

strength has declined compared to the rest of my body. I want to balance them now, the upper part with the lower part.

We could ask: which *balance* would Pedro be talking about? *What upper part or lower part is he talking about?* Pedro reveals an idea of the self in pieces—in parts that cannot come together and cannot produce a whole. He hasn't developed a language to connect his body with his mind.

In this paper, I investigate the role of the body in primordial mental states. I develop ideas about the functioning of the primordial mind and consider that the body in these states is an "inhabited body" (Maiello, 2011), one uninhabited by a self. I examine the language used by the analyst to help the patient in becoming a body, "being a body", and connecting his body to his mind. I propose that this language should be what I call a "language of emotion" (Korbivcher, 2020). Pedro's clinical material will be presented to illustrate these ideas and open the topic for discussion.

Primordial mind

In his clinical practice, the psychoanalyst must ask himself, with each movement in the session, who the patient he is meeting with is, and at what mental level he is operating—whether it is on a neurotic or psychotic level, or rather if it is on a primordial level and therefore autistic and unintegrated. The answer to this question is a crucial one since the rules that operate on neurotic or psychotic levels are completely different from those that operate on primordial levels.

Freud (1923) pointed out the continuity between pre and postnatal life stating, "there is much more continuity between intrauterine life and earliest infancy than the impressive caesura of the act of birth would have us believe" (p. 138). This statement by Freud began a now wide-ranging field of investigation into pre-natal psychism in contemporary psychoanalysis.

In his later works, Bion (1976a to 1992) showed great interest in the functioning of the embryonic mental states and primordial mental phenomena, as well as their effects on post-natal infant communications and their relations. For Bion, the primordial mind is the starting point of psychic activity.

Bion (1977) in Caesura asks:

Is it possible for us, as psycho-analysts, to think that there may still be vestiges in the human being that would suggest a survival in the human mind, analogous to that in the human body, of evidence in the field of optics that once there were optic pits, or in the field of hearing that once there were auditory pits? Is there any part of the human mind which still betrays signs of an 'embryological' intuition, either visual or auditory?

(p. 44)

Bion relates the primordial mind to a type of imaginary embryology of the mind. For him, the mental equivalents of embryonic remnants are apparent even in civilized and cultured individuals who exercise the more developed function of speech. He suggests that the pre-natal sensations could be the origin of proto emotions, including states of subthalamic terror. This type of fear isn't controlled by the mind, and it therefore doesn't acquire meaning. It is expressed by intense bodily manifestations of remnants of prenatal parts, involving the adrenal glands and adrenaline secretion, which are activated at certain moments (Braga & Korbivcher, 2018).

As Bion (1979) said, "the nearest he can get to giving it a provisional title, is the *inaccessible state of mind*".

For Green, the term "primordial mind" is based on its opposition to the "civilized, individual, educated, and articulated" parts of the human being.

Green (1998) writes,

> Bion relates the primordial mind to some sort of imaginary embryology of the mind. He shares a common hypothesis with Freud that there is something primitive in the mind that is not entirely explained by the early stages of object relationships in the development of the baby. The traces left by phylogenesis and ontogenesis in the structure of the mind should play a significant role in later stages of development.
>
> (p. 651)

Green goes on to ask:

> The primordial mind is made up of thoughts which, because of their raw and crude nature, are not workable as such. So, they must be expelled from the psyche.... How can a thought without a thinker be expelled from the mind, considering that the discharge process sends them out of the mind and does not carry with it the whole of the primitive mental activity? The probable answer is that it is impossible to get rid entirely of the β-elements that stay blocked in the mind and will poison other mental processes if they gain the upper hand again.
>
> (p. 651)

This means that the mind contains unborn embryonic remnants that have not been transformed, and that remain present even in the minds of neurotic individuals throughout their lives. Bion's emphasis on the primordial mind favors the individual recognizing these manifestations without representation, navigating through them, and eventually transforming them into something meaningful, that can be thought and named.

One of the fundamental discoveries of psychoanalysis, according to Bion, would be contact with these archaic mental states, and with primitive patterns of behavior that can be detected even in the most civilized and cultured individuals (Bion, 1977, p. 53).

But his question remains: "how could we penetrate the caesura of birth?" (Bion, 1977). For the analyst working at this level, the crucial point in practice is how to traverse the caesura that separates the pre- and post-natal universes and establish a communication between these two worlds.

Manifestations of these archaic mental states can be identified (Bion, 1981) by the analyst, by their characteristics: "being alone and dependent", "urge to exist", and "primitive moral conscience"[2] (Junqueira de Mattos & Braga, 2013; Braga & Korbivcher, 2018).

In clinical practice primordial mental states can be recognized by the presence of autistic transformations and unintegrated transformations (Korbivcher, 2014, 2017).[3] When these transformations are present, the analyst is tasked to provide language establishing communication with the patient at the level of his primordial mind, assisting him to establish contact between his body and mind, between sensations and the psyche, and eventually in creating an inner self that inhabits his body.

The body

As Freud (1923) states, "at the beginning of life the ego is first and foremost a body ego". This means that from the beginning, the individual has a sense of identity that derives from the consciousness that he has a body, that he is that body, and that this body has some perception of itself. This awareness also allows him to recognize the presence of a separate other and thus begin to establish relations (Maiello, 2011).

Maiello (2011) writes:

> It is difficult to imagine a living body without an even fleeting awareness of itself. *Being* one's body and *knowing about* being that body seems to be at the core of the sense of identity and of the capacity to relate to other living beings.

This suggests that every living body has a short-lived consciousness of existence since very early in life. This consciousness is developed through the individual relationship to his own body by the notion of *having a body,* and of *being that body*.

At the initial stage of life according to Winnicott (1945), integration is as important as the development of feeling what is inside one's own body. For him, human nature is psychosomatic: psyche and soma tend to progressively integrate themselves into a unit in such a way that the psyche is felt to reside in the body. For this to occur, as Winnicott states, "there must be a living and continuous presence of someone to hold and care for the infant, providing it the experience of being together through a mother's look and being in her arms" (Winnicott, 1988, p. 29). We can suppose that with this experience an intimate connection is established between soma and psyche, the psyche now lodging itself in the body.

Following along in the same direction, Bick (1968, 1986) introduces the notion of the "psychic skin" as one of the rudiments of the notion of self. She states that it is from the introjection of an external object, interacting continuously with the surface of the infant's body, that a psychic skin will be formed, allowing then for developmental movement toward fantasies about internal and external space. She goes on to say that—should this process fail for any reason—a second skin with autistic characteristics will be formed to protect the infant from intolerable unintegrated experiences. The threat of falling into an endless space, of dissolving, and spilling are expressions of these unintegrated states. That is, the threat of losing the notion of one's own existence (Bick, 1968; Tustin, 1992).

Patients operating in autistic states relate by adhesiveness (Meltzer 1975; Bick 1986), in two-dimensional ways in which there is no space between self and object, and no notion of possessing an interior or an exterior. The individual in these states entertains, through auto sensuous activities, experiences of continuity with the object, avoiding intolerable feelings of terror when faced with the awareness of bodily separation. For him, the body corresponds to a pathological exoskeleton, without containing an endoskeleton in his interior that would convey a sense of psychic existence. In Maiello's terms, this is an "uninhabited body".

For Maiello, *being one's body* and *having a body* are linked to the awareness of inhabiting one's body, an awareness which allows the individual to develop a sense of otherness. Maiello (2011) asks:

> What is the experience that can be expected of an autistic child to have of his own body, if there is no subject, no ego capable of experiencing himself or herself as an I and therefore of the body *as my body*?

We can say then, along with Maiello, that an autistic child experiences his body as a "no-body", of not *being a body*. It is a flat body with no volume and without a definite shape, with no delimitation, that spreads out in pieces, in parts that do not put themselves together. To obtain a cohesive state, the child adheres to another body, or remains withdrawn into the interior of a protective shell absorbed by autosensuous *activities*.

Pedro

Pedro is 20 years old and has been in analysis for several years, three times a week. He sought out analysis because it is difficult for him to connect with people. He recoils into his own world most of the time, closing himself off in his room where he spends hours listening to music or watching movies on his iPad. Pedro also mentions that he feels frustrated at not being able to date girls because as he says, after kissing a girl at a party, he is unable to maintain a conversation with her.

Pedro is a tall and handsome young man. His gaze is distant and rather inexpressive. He seems burdened by having to carry the enormous weight of his own body. His voice is low and very deep, his speech is monotonous, and without any kind of affective modulation.

Pedro's current focus in his sessions revolves mainly around his body and exercising at the gym.

Upon calling Pedro for his session, I find him on his iPhone, his attention rapt and wearing headphones. When he sees me, he quickly removes the headphones and stands up, extending a limp handshake, throwing a fleeting glance my way and greeting me with a nod. He walks toward our room with a kind of disjointed gait, lies down, and—just as in many of our sessions—quickly, quietly, and inwardly asks, "What's up?"

I respond emphatically asking him: "What's UP there?"

He stays silent for a long time. Then I question him about what he is thinking. Pedro speaks in his usual deep, monotone, and emotionless voice—a voice that makes it difficult to deduce the message that he wishes to convey, and as if he were talking to himself. He says that he was thinking about his exercise plan for the week, that he was thinking about adding more leg exercises because he thinks his legs are too weak and thin.

He says, *"I want to work on my strength to improve my volleyball game, to get healthier. I used to only want to get bigger, stronger. I thought more about my looks, and I didn't work out my legs. I've had a good workout with my upper body and my legs got weaker in comparison to the rest of my body. Now I want to balance the upper half a little better with the lower half"*.

I follow this concrete speech about his legs, arms, and lower parts, within a scattered and rather emotionless mental state. I hear unarticulated sounds without any emotional involvement. Suddenly I awaken from this state and realize that Pedro, in his way, is presenting me with his self-image ... a body in pieces, without a "self" that inhabits its interior. I share the approximate meaning of this idea with him.

He says, "If I could balance all of this, one part would be able to help the other".

He dives again into a long silence ... I feel isolated, without an interlocutor with whom to communicate. I notice a tendency to retreat into my own thoughts and giving up on making contact with him. However, when I recognize this, I regain my analytic functioning, and I invite him back to our communication. Otherwise, we would both have remained in our current states.

I tell him that he might not only be talking about arms and legs, but that he also appears not to have found the balance inside himself that will give him some internal support and direction on how to communicate with me. I say that he is talking about the balance in his body, between the upper part, and the lower part, but I ask if the balance that he is looking for might not be that between his body and his mind...

He is surprised and somewhat perplexed, asking, "How is that? Is it emotion?" After some time, he says thoughtfully, "I think that my emotion is linked to my body because after I work out, I look at myself in the mirror and feel satisfied, in a good mood when I see my body..."

I reply that perhaps for him the exercises give him the idea of having some contour around his body, which provides him the sensation of having at least a physical existence, like this one that he sees in the mirror.

At this moment, I notice a change in our previously stalled, emotionless atmosphere. He appears to be more present, and alive.

He says,

> I think that my embarrassment when speaking, when I start to speak, improved because of the way I see myself physically. This takes away my embarrassment. When people talk about politics, I feel a little stupid ... but, in general, after this physical change, I am feeling a little more secure.

I tell him that maybe some things have been put together inside of him during our conversation, giving him more confidence to communicate. He states that lately he has been more confident to put himself out there, instead of passing himself off as invisible, as he had sometimes done during college when he would sit in the back of the classroom, looking at the ground and not looking forward. He says that now he is looking forward, making eye contact with those coming in the opposite direction, and is present even when he does not have anything to say.

I feel touched by his suffering when faced with the terror caused by the awareness of the separate other, and the maneuvers he must carry out to confront this situation. I share this idea and add that he speaks through his body that which he deals with internally. I add that he feels like those pieces are all spread out around him; the upper part, the lower part, legs, and arms do not give him the idea that he has his own existence. There are only pieces, scattered parts.

He replies,

> Yes! The more pieces there are, the more embarrassed I feel. It's hard to quantify these emotional things. With the body image it's easier. We can see the changes in everything—in the physical and the emotional. I feel more satisfied recently, with my performance. I can see an improvement!

I remark that it appears that throughout the session he has stopped being invisible like he was in the beginning. At first, he started talking about his gym exercises, getting stronger, the upper part and the lower. But as we talked his mind started to emerge, and he felt more of a balance between mind and body, with a sense of himself looking in the mirror and seeing the contour of a person satisfied by seeing his own image.

I notice him to be enthusiastic, more alive, curious, and showing more emotion than I had ever observed before.

Pedro continues,

> Another thing I can observe about the physical and the emotional is that I used to think I couldn't increase my very thin physique. I thought I would always be shy in any situation; I quickly gave up on talking. This perception has also changed; I thought I don't have to keep being shy. Now I have the desire to assert myself. I thought that I would always be this way ... but now I see that it can be different.

I say, "For someone who said that he didn't have anything to say today ... how does this conversation feel to you?"

He replies "At first I was feeling more reserved as in yesterday's session. Now that has changed. I'm not as hesitant. Today the conversation was more fluid, more direct".

I tell him that he is indeed present, not needing to hide himself or remain invisible.

The session ends. Pedro gets up and shakes my hand somewhat firmly. He looks me in the eye, gives me the hint of a smile, and leaves.

Comments

Pedro's functioning displays many characteristics of the primordial mind. He manifests important autistic barriers. His gaze, emotionless and distant, the limp hands, low tone of voice, in addition to his silence and reclusion in the sessions, are suggestive of this state. The long, greasy hair covering his face reminds one of a mask protecting him from the presence of the other. Pedro seeks refuge in his shelter, distancing himself from the human world, which means that he does not develop resources for sharing experiences with others.

In the session described, upon meeting the analyst, Pedro puts his ritual into action—extending a feeble hand and his usual question: "What's up?" He appeals to these autistic maneuvers with the intention of protecting himself from the threats experienced when faced with the presence of the analyst as a separate person.

After waiting for a while, the analyst invites him to communicate. He quickly speaks about increasing the amount of exercise for his body. He speaks about a body in pieces, with parts that do not come together: legs, disarticulated arms, the upper part, the lower part. He speaks about a lack of balance in his body. With the concrete nature of this narrative and the lack of emotion, the analyst leans toward evasion until she can recover her role and give meaning to what she is witnessing: the description of Pedro's self-image, the self as a recipient, as pieces unable to find balance between the parts, or sustain them.

Pedro presents pain at the awareness of this condition and tries to reunite the pieces to obtain balance, or rather, to gain support. The analyst is emotionally touched by this scenario and, being at one with Pedro's mental state, invites him to abandon his autistic refuge and share with her his discomfort, his pain.

Pedro feels contained by the analyst and he becomes more alive and curious. This gives him the experience of having a contour for his body—his body image reflected in the mirror. The analyst suggests to him that the balance he seeks could be between his mind and his body. This formulation stimulates Pedro's thinking, allowing him to conceive at that point the beginnings of a self to inhabit his body. At the end of the session, Pedro stops being invisible and is stimulated to be in better contact with the analyst.

Discussion

Pedro is clear in revealing what an uninhabited body means: legs, arms, upper part, lower part, without a balance between the parts, or rather, without a balance between mind and body. It is a body in pieces without an interior self that can recognize otherness.

It remains a question: how can the analyst provide Pedro *a balance between the upper part with the lower part,* or contact between mind and body, or, in Pedro's own words, the contact between *body and emotion*? How can the analyst "penetrate the caesura of birth" (Bion, 1977)?

As we can see, Pedro has not developed an inner self to sustain him when confronting separateness from the object and this causes him to experience states of extreme vulnerability. He protects himself, withdrawing into his inanimate world where he becomes invisible and insensitive. He is enough for himself, avoiding therefore feelings of helplessness when faced with otherness.

The body is his primary means of communication. It is through his uninhabited body that he expresses what he is dealing with. Pedro developed a pathological exoskeleton, pathological because it contained no endoskeleton. Had there been an endoskeleton it would have provided him with the notion of having an interior existence. Instead, he depends on adhesivity to the object as a way of obtaining some cohesion through the sensation of continuity and a sense of existence at the body level.

Pedro shows a discrepancy between his adolescent body and the Pedro/inhabited body. He cannot bear the body's normative sexual demands of adolescence, lacking a corresponding emotional dimension to accompany them. He complains that he can't build on his encounters with girls, which begin as sexualized exchanges. He feels that he cannot find an internal mental counterpart capable of sustaining the situation.

The analyst, being in unison with Pedro's mental state—a body split into separate pieces—tries to reunite these pieces by inviting him to share his pain with her. She mentions that Pedro was maybe not only interested in legs and arms, but was also looking for some internal support to sustain all these pieces together, a *balance* between his mind and his body. At this moment, Pedro's state of mind changes. He becomes attracted by this formulation and astonished, he asks, "*What is this? Is this emotion?*"

I suggest that what first attracted Pedro to make contact was the analyst's emotion, expressed by the modulation of her voice and through her facial expression, but not by the content of her words. This is what I am calling a "language of emotion" (Korbivcher, 2020). The analyst, through being at one with the patient's mental state, becomes the emotion of the moment.

Pedro inquisitively mentions that he feels emotion when looking at the image of his own body in a mirror at the gym and is happy with what he sees. I understand that Pedro at this moment could see the shape of his image reflected in the analyst's look, an image of his "body-self". His image, as he said, pleases him. Pedro at this point is stimulated to consider the origins of a mind emerging from this uninhabited body. He stops being invisible in the session, becoming more alive and interested in the contact with the analyst.

We can suppose that this was the beginning of the development of a language between Pedro's body and his mind. Pedro "being a body"—this is the balance that he was seeking in this session.

Our challenge as psychoanalysts working with patients like Pedro is to help them constitute a mind which inhabits their bodies, in a way that the yet unborn primordial mental elements become psychic elements which would eventually be transformed into thoughts and emotions. Our aim is to establish a communication between "what is buried in a forgotten past or in a becoming future" (Bion, 1977, p. 125). In other words, establishing a communication between unborn life and post-natal life.

Notes

1 Maiello (2020).
2 Bion & Bion (1981), in a key to *A Memoir of the Future*, write: "Be dependent and alone: it seems to me that even a baby—although it can't verbalize it, of course—feels dependent and feels all alone" (p. 25). The urge to exist: "The impulse to exist is postulated even as an urge to which the individual is 'slave'..." (p. 31). Primitive moral conscience: "Its basic characteristic is being always ready to say what we should not do or think, but never what we should do. The idea is of a 'feeling of guilt' which someday turns into a kind of conscience".
3 Unintegrated transformations occur in an unintegrated medium. They can be identified by the presence of intense un-mentalized corporeal manifestations, without psychic representation. Their invariants are a constant state of terror that comes from experiencing the threat of falling into an endless abyss, dilution, and

dissolution—in other words, the loss of notion of one's own existence (Korbivcher, 2017). Autistic transformations form themselves in an autistic medium, which implies the absence of notion of an external or internal object. Their invariants are the presence of self-sensory activities, the absence of affective life, the experience of an affective void. The relations between the "self" and "non-self" occur through sensation objects—objects and autistic shapes (Korbivcher, 2014).

References

Bick, E. (1968). The experience of the skin in early object-relations. *International Journal of Psychoanalysis*, 49, 484–486.

Bick, E. (1986). Further considerations on the function of the skin in early object relations: Findings from infant observation integrated into child and adult analysis. *Brit. J. Psychotherapy*, 2(4), 292–299.

Bion, R.W. (1976a/1987). Emotional turbulence. In *Clinical seminars and four papers*. Fleetwood Press.

Bion, R.W. (1976b/1987). Evidence. In *Clinical seminars and four papers*. Fleetwood Press.

Bion, R.W. (1977 [1975]). *Two papers: The grid and caesura*. Ed. Imago.

Bion, R.W. (1979/1987). Making the best of a bad job. In *Clinical seminars and four papers*. Fleetwood Press.

Bion, R.W., & Bion, F. (1981). *A key to a memoir of the future*. Clunie Press.

Bion, R.W. (1991). *A memoir of the future*. Ed. Karnac.

Bion, R.W. (1992). *Taming wild thoughts*. Karnac.

Braga, J.C., & Korbivcher, C.F. (2018). Bion: A Mente Primordial e a Clinica. Um ou Quatro Modelos de Funcionamento Mental? [The primordial mind and practice. One or four models of mental functioning?] (Unpublished).

Freud, S. (1923). O Ego e o Id [The ego and the id]. In *Obras Completas Brasileiras [Full Brazilian Works]* (Vol. XIX).

Green, A. (1998). The primordial mind and the work of the negative. *Int. J. Psychoanal.*, 79(4), 649–665.

Junqueira de Mattos, J.A., & Braga, J.C. (2013). Primitive conscience: A glimpse of the primordial mind. In H.B. Levine & L.J. Brown (Eds.), *Growth and turbulence in the container/contained – Bion's continuing legacy*. Routledge.

Korbivcher, C.F. (2014). The theory of transformations and autistic states. Autistic transformations a proposal. In *Autistic transformations: Bion's theory and autistic phenomena*. Karnac Books.

Korbivcher, C.F. (2017). Bion and unintegrated states. Falling dissolving and spilling. In H. Levine & D. Power (Eds.), *Engaging primitive anxieties of the emerging self. The legacy of Frances Tustin*. Karnac.

Korbivcher, C.F. (2020). A Mente Primordial e a Linguagem do Analista: uma linguagem de emoção [The primordial mind and analyst language: A language of emotion]. *Rev. Bras de Psicanálise*, 54(3).

Maiello, S. (2011). Psychoanalytic considerations on the uninhabited body of the autistic child. In Conference in Autistic Spectrun desorder II at the Brazilian Psychoanalytic Society of São Paulo, 27 November 2014. Also in: *Journal de la Psychanalyse de L'enfant*, 1, 109–139.

Maiello, S. (2020). *On the absence of bodily awareness in autistic children*. Frances Tustin Lectureship Day, 06 November 2020.

Meltzer, D. (1975/1986). Identificação adesiva [Adhesive identification]. *Jornal de Psicanálise Ano*, 19(38).

Tustin, F. (1992). *Autistic states in children* (revised edition). Routledge.

Winnicott, D. (1945). Desenvolvimento emocional primitivo. In D.W. Winnicott, *Da pediatria à psicanálise: obras escolhidas* (2000, pp. 218–232), Trans. D. Bogomoletz. Imago.

Winnicott, D. (1988). *Human nature*. Free Association Books.

Chapter 9

Perceptual identification as analytic receptivity of unrepresented and dissociative states

Judy K. Eekhoff

Analytic reverie is severely challenged when working with patients who have suffered early accumulated trauma—that is childhood trauma that was an aspect of their everyday lives from birth to emancipation from their families. Often these are the patients who come to us with life-long pain and frustration, but seemingly without feeling much of their childhood trauma. They can tell us many stories. They *know* they had a difficult childhood, but seemingly they have not *suffered* their pain (Bion, 1970). They have used primary dissociation, that is, separating their bodies from their minds (Bion, 1967; Lombardi, 2017; Goldberg, 2021; Eekhoff, 2022), to escape the pain and frustrations of their abuse. Primary dissociation involves precocious mental development that forecloses mind body cohesion and integration. Their emotions are also much reduced in that they seem unable to express or feel them. Sometimes they know this. Sometimes they do not. Often, they tell us something is missing in them. Sometimes they tell us they cannot love. More often still, they tell us they feel isolated, but are most comfortable being alone.

Goldberg (2021) describes what he calls *beta function*, the ongoing not-ever-to-be-represented body as background object. Although I would not use the words beta functioning, I believe he is describing a very important element of what it is to be embodied and the pleasure the body brings. In this chapter, I am focusing on the opposite of that: diffusion of the self and a defensive foregrounding of sensation that occurs in response to trauma. In using the body and the senses as defense, pleasure is lost as is a capacity for intimacy. Lack of representation is also both defensive and the result of an external attack that overrode the apparatus for thinking and interfered with its development. Without the capacities to represent relationship, complexity and depth of that which was experienced are lost (Bion, 1965). Lost also are the capacities to love and to grieve the loss of a love. As one patient asked me, "How I do I grieve something I have never had?" For these patients, primal dissociation of severing the body mind union is more prevalent than is dissociation via splitting and projective identification or repression. Each of these require an object. Primary dissociation forecloses the possibility of an

DOI: 10.4324/9781003534365-9

internal containing object and in doing so forecloses further development of a subjective sense of self.

For me, this dissociation occurring in infancy involves dispersal of the self via excessive splitting and projection into infinity instead of projection into an object (Eekhoff, 2022, pp. 5–6). States of primary undifferentiation result. They appear to be primary narcissism, something neither Klein nor I believe in. Rather these undifferentiated states are defensive and the result of an overwhelming traumatic experience. Undifferentiation is accomplished by dissociation of body and mind during which the mind becomes more important than the body, hence initiating precocious mental development that includes a premature cruel superego. Auto-sensuous defenses separate the person from his or her objects, reinforcing an unconscious phantasy of no objects available. Since trauma survivors use primal dissociation and primary undifferentiation as extra-ordinary protections (Mitrani, 2001), they also suffer from unmentalized states and unrepresented states. These are present, not as holding and containing background objects, but as an *unthought known* (Bollas, 1987) that persecutes.

When an adult patient seems to have primitive states wherein there is little differentiation between the internal world and the external world, chaos and violence reigns. As infants this lack of differentiation is more comfortable, especially if there is a good enough background of safety provided by the caregivers. In dissociating in order to survive their childhoods, these adults limit their possibility for growth and development. For as Bion (1970) says, "the patient who will not suffer pain fails to 'suffer' pleasure and this denies the patient the encouragement he might otherwise receive from accidental or intrinsic relief" (p. 9). Since projective identification can be a means of communicating and receiving help in dealing with unprocessed pain, it is an important part of coping with difficult circumstances. We know he also says that projective identification is the foundation for thinking and that it can be disrupted, thus disturbing the development of thinking itself. He says,

> In some patients the denial to the patient of a normal employment of projective identification precipitates a disaster through the destruction of an important link. Inherent in this disaster is the establishment of a primitive superego which denies the use of projective identification.
>
> (1958, p. 146)

When parents are the cause of accumulated childhood trauma, they are denying their children the use of themselves as receptors of projective identifications. Their children cannot communicate their pain, even unconsciously via projective identification. This ultimately disrupts these projective and introjective processes. Children subsequently develop premature superegos and internalize obstructive objects (Bion, 1958; Skogstad, 2013). Bion (1967) says they prematurely become aware of their own personalities.

I use prenatal and postnatal infantile experience as a model for the work we do with these patients. I do not equate the adult with the infant or even attempt to have the patient regress to infancy. That infancy is always present in the hour. Again, quoting Bion (1992),

> Winnicott says patients need to regress: Melanie Klein says they must not: I say they are regressed, and the regression should be observed and interpreted by the analyst without any need to compel the patient to become totally regressed before he can make the analyst observe and interpret the regression.
>
> (p. 166)

For me, this implies that an analyst will be able to use reverie as a means of anticipating a patient's response to an interpretation. This is not necessarily via the reception of projective identifications, rather may come through adhesive identifications. This requires the analyst's unconscious use of perceptual identification.

Sometimes the unconscious-to-unconscious reception occurs via reverberations or resonances that are discovered in the body of the analyst. These impressions present as somatic counter-transference. These are derivatives of impressions or traces of experience that have not been mentalized. However, I also believe that not every analysand/analyst dyad is a good fit for each member.

In health, the mother's love for her unborn and newly born infant is communicated via her reverie. Her joy, passion, and awe at the mystery of life invokes representation and a rich mental life in her infant. It impacts the infant's growing ability to dream meaning into experience (Monteiro, 2023, p. 128). I believe infants are born object related even though their primary mode of relating is body relations. During nursing the infant is taking in the body relations and the object relations of its mother. Along with milk comes the mother's love or hate, and it is this emotional link that enables the infant's mind to be called forth in a healthy relational manner.

Trauma disrupts this process and object relations. Traumatized infants and children retreat to their bodies as defense. Their body relations are proximate and sensual, without bringing pleasure; sensations and sensory perceptions dominate as defense. This results in a loss of the object and inhibition of introjection. Without awareness of the other, the budding subjective sense of self is also delayed. The primal dissociation of body and mind protects these trauma survivors from awareness of being projected into and not received.

With accumulated childhood trauma, both the mental apparatus for processing relationships and the emotional complexity of being human is compromised. This means that projective and introjective processes that are the foundation for future thinking become inadequate. As Bion (1965) says, "the growth of insight depends, at its inception, on undisturbed functioning of projective identification" (p. 36). Patients who were abused as young children and who use primal dissociation and undifferentiation as defenses have retreated from parents who seemingly were *obstructive objects* (Bion, 1958)—that is, they did not often enough receive their infant's projective identifications through their reverie. Bion (1970) says the way a mother shows her love for her infant is by reverie: "when a mother loves the infant what does she do it with? Leaving aside the physical channels of communication my impression is that her love is expressed by reverie" (pp. 35–36).

An analyst working with a person who does not always split and project and then re-introject with proficiency faces challenges to his or her imaginative conjecture, receptive openness, and even the unconscious communication such processes promote. Reverie in the face of a psychically absent other, such as the primally dissociative patient I am describing, is difficult. Without receiving the expected emotional contact from the patient in the form of projective identifications, interpreting the transference can become a mental activity, not one of intuitive understanding. This is a repetition of the primal dissociation of the patient and evidence of an obstructive internal object in the analyst who does not notice the lack of connection and/or in the patient who bounces the analyst's projective-identification-as-communication back. The obstructive object can be in either the patient or the analyst or both.

In instances where projective processes are damaged, I believe we do the best we can, using our reverie and our openness to "find" the person with us. Bergstein (2019, p. 39) quotes Meltzer: "in these unmentalized states, the analyst 'must be capable of imaginative thought, or dream-thought, that embraces the intra-uterine experience as a "world" quite different from the "world" of projective identification' (Meltzer, 1986, p. 36)". The world these patients bring us is a world we must enter if we are to be of service. This is a world of body relations, of synchrony and rhythmicity, of sound and sensation. It is a world of music and dance. It is a mysterious world outside of the symbolic order.

When our receptivity and openness, important analytic values, are met with indifference and seemingly little response, we can fall back upon Bion's belief that

> Receptiveness achieved by denudation of memory and desire (which is essential to the operation of 'acts of faith') is essential to the operation of psycho-analysis and other scientific proceedings. It is essential for experiencing hallucination or the state of hallucinosis.
>
> (1970, pp. 35–36)

Hallucinosis is an aspect of everyday analytic work (Civitarese, 2012, 2015). However, analysts often find such a state uncomfortable and threatening, since it can evoke a feeling of not existing psychically for themselves or for the patient. Included in this may be the analyst's own defensive blockage of psychic aliveness.

When it seems we do not psychically exist for our patients, our own narcissistic needs to exist interfere with disciplined stances of no memory and desire. Mind takes over and analysts can be drawn into thinking too much. Such thinking interferes with reverie. For example, when this happens to me, I find myself thinking about theory or watch myself observing and mentally describing what is happening. I talk to myself, "Remember this. What is happening here?" These side trips away from my patient are important means of holding myself, but that is the point. They are not the result of my receptivity of unconscious communication, or of projective identification, or even of psychic deadness coming from my patient—not that all those things do not also happen. Such "side trips" are not a reverie to be used for understanding my patient. However, they are a hallucinosis—a state where I become my dissociated patient and am no longer embodied. I then become an obstructive object.

There can be words coming from both patient and analyst. Sometimes there are too many words. Words can be used as shields, sounds not to be interpreted for their content but for their auto-sensuous function of protection. Some of these words are more than mimicry or self-soothing, but finding the symbols of truth beneath the mimicry and self-soothing can be difficult. Sifting through the debris and sounds of words might put the analyst into an experience of being the patient.

Again, for me such an experience is terrifying because, at once, I am witness to my patient's self-annihilation even as I myself am being obliterated. Further, this symbiosis seems to happen in the presence of the other without effort, passively. At the most primal level, symbiosis does not include violence or attacks on the psyche. It occurs via bodily proximity, even on screen. It is in the sensual link, the symbiotic link between patient and analyst. Hence it is the arena of perceptual identity and primary process. Symbiosis is a foundational experience, found in all of us (Bleger, 1967), however it can and is also used defensively.

One could say analytic symbiosis is akin to maternal preoccupation, but not quite. It is outside of awareness until it can be gathered and slowly over time named and described. This is the bodily gathering of the transference (Meltzer, 1986). Goldberg (2021) believes that some of these bodily sensations are never to be named—but serve as beta functions—like a backdrop to the self. My language for this is slightly different, but if I understand him correctly, this arena of the self—undifferentiated and undrawn, but none-the-less present is backdrop for us all. I believe Bleger (1967) is also exploring this primal position of the self, which is a body relation filled with sensuous pleasure in the physical sound and sensation of another. That is the healthy aspect.

Rather now, I am writing about, trying to find words for, a primal dissociative state of nonexistence that includes few represented and few projected states. It is the arena of experience of the *unrepressed unconscious*. If the unconscious is conscious (Bion, 1970; Bergstein, 2019), without a repression barrier or a contact barrier as protection, there is no need for projection. There is also little opportunity to use projective identification as a means of communication because undifferentiation between self and other wipes out an object to project into. Without an object, the projection into the universe that occurs can only be used to rid the psyche of debris. The primal dissociative state becomes a background of the self and what is presented is behavior without true relationship. If I am correct, this helps us understand the force that keeps trauma alive year after year, without seeming diminishment.

When patients have withdrawn so far into themselves or exploded into infinite space, it is very hard to be with them. It is difficult to be open and receptive to the nothingness of mindless states. This is true especially when the patient is able to present a false self or an as-if self of mimicry. I believe that whereas patience and non-intrusiveness are extremely important, so too is calling a patient forth, saying "Come, come" (Eekhoff, 2019, 2022) or "Hey, there" (Alvarez, 1992). This is done by remaining in the here and now with the mystery and awe of getting to know this other person and being actively engaged.

Clinical example

Let me tell you of a patient and my attempts to find him. I have written of him before (Eekhoff, 2022) as an example of primal hope. Of course, this story that I tell of him does not begin to convey the truth of our meetings. There was so much more than anything I might say. The mystery and depth of our work cannot be described.

Dennis is now in his eighties. He came to me when he was seventy-four. Initially, I was not sure why he came. His attempts to describe his need for a second analysis were vague. I registered his ambivalence: he told me he had called me several times in the past ten years, listening to my voice but not leaving a message. He said my voice was "too deep". After our first visit, he asked for a referral, telling me "You are too far away". A month later, he returned, saying he wanted to work with me. He was a pleasant, well-groomed man who seemingly engaged easily. Since he was retired from a good job, he felt he had time to get to know himself better.

Dennis was college educated but reported, "It took me a few extra years because I had difficulty remembering things and I couldn't think". As with everything else he told me in these beginning years, his voice was calm and matter-of-fact. He reported without feeling. He told me he decided to come now, "because my cat died". He had had a previous ten-year experience in college with analytic group therapy. This ended when the analyst died. Later he had a nine-year analysis as well as a ten-year live-in relationship with a man who died of AIDS. He reported without feeling although he described both of these later relationships as bad for him. I noticed that he seemed to almost equate his former analyst with his live-in partner. We began at once a week, soon moved to twice a week and then to three times a week. He did not use the couch, "because I don't like women".

I began to fear the work we were doing, since I imagined he would suffer greatly if we connected deeply and emotionally, as is usual in analysis. This fear of mine, I believe, was the first evidence that he was beginning to project into me and to make use of me. But I worried. Would analysis only make him suffer? Would he die before our work was finished? He was so determined to be "better", but I did not think he knew what that would require.

I learned that Dennis was an unwelcome child (Ferenczi, 1929; Eekhoff, 2022). He was the fourth child and the third boy. Purportedly, according to family myth, his mother wanted another girl and thrust the infant back at the nurses with disgust, telling them to keep him. Three other children followed—all girls. The home he was born into was not a happy one. His parents fought continually, and the children were frequent victims of physical and emotional abuse. Much later, he told me several of his sisters had accused their father of sexual abuse. He didn't know if it was true or not, but concluded anything was possible in that house. Dennis described his childhood home as a "house of horrors". He did not bring friends there.

School was escape for him, but he did not do particularly well. He said he always had trouble concentrating and lived in a dream world. He focused on having friends, many of them girls. He also took refuge at his grandmother's house who claimed him as her favorite. In spite of seemingly being a "good boy", he described getting beaten by both parents. I did not ask for these stories. They were part of the script Dennis believed every analyst wanted.

When I remarked on our process, he would sometimes look confused. He told me I talked more than his first analyst did, which made him doubt our work was anything but social. He regretted that he had used the couch or stayed so long with his former analyst. He did not want to make the same mistake with me. He described being paranoid and obsessive, because his first analyst had told him he was. Apparently, he had also been told that there was no treatment for either paranoia or obsessiveness.

When I attempted to interpret the transference, he would continue talking as if I had said nothing. If I commented, he would say, "This isn't about you". When I said he seemed to want me to know all of his history, he said his first analyst did. If I attempted to add to what he was saying, he would say, "I didn't say that". There was no rancor in his voice. He was merely stating the fact. He seemed to have no idea two analysts were not the same or that a conversation could build on itself, with each participant contributing and elaborating an idea or a feeling. I began to think that he was not in relationship with me because there was really only room for one of us. Should he become aware of me, I could only become identified as an aggressor (Ferenczi, 1933). This would interfere with his purpose.

I am not sure how long it took me to recognize that when I spoke, he would dissociate. The difficulty was that if I didn't, he would dissociate too. Silences were difficult for him because he told me he fell into "mindless places". Previously (Eekhoff, 2022), I described him as blinking on and off like Christmas tree lights, but this coming and going was not splitting. Rather it was what Ferenczi (1933) has called *atomization.* He was dissolving or evaporating in front of me and seemingly without form. In those moments, he was experiencing *"objectless sensation"* (Ferenczi, 1955) as well as an *inhibited attempt at splitting* (ibid.). He con-formed with me, taking shape via the setting of my office (Bleger, 1967). He began to speak about my office, describing it and missing it when he was not there. He said, *"When I am in your room, I feel I am in my lower garden where I have room to feel these things".* When I said he equated my office with me, he just looked at me, blinking. After a while he said, *"Maybe".* Today, I might say he equated my office with his garden, alive. He did not seem to equate my office with me. I was not yet a person to him.

He displayed little agency and seemed extremely passive. His primary activity other than his analysis was working out 3 or 4 hours a day at a local gym. He also continued to read his many books on psychoanalysis and to talk to me about Karen Horney. Once he said, "You know you look like her, don't you?". Another time he described listening to her on You Tube and told me "You sound like her". Here again we have evidence of equating two people in an almost hallucinatory manner.

As I began to experience his dissociation, I felt increasingly upset by it. I could never be sure if he heard me or registered even my presence, although he watched me intensely. On the one hand, he appeared alert, almost hyper-vigilant and hyper-sensitive to changes in the frame. On the other, he appeared indifferent and very young, almost newborn or even unborn. Sometimes, his rapid blinking would turn into a stare. I began intuitively to describe what was happening in the room, in the atmosphere, so to speak. Whenever I told him it was time to end our session, he would abruptly rise and exit, without looking back.

Once when Seattle suffered a major snow-storm, he came anyway in spite of his fear of driving. Later, I went outside to get the mail, and discovered someone had shoveled my sidewalk and driveway. It was he.

There are many things I could say about Dennis, but I want to focus on an important aspect of our work together. Our relationship was seemingly devoid of feeling. I found working with him pleasant, but not initially stimulating. I also did not feel as if I "received" any projections from him. Nor was I bored or sleepy or even confused. I was mildly curious as to why he was with me. In the initial stage, it seemed he was repeating what he had told his previous analysts.

Slowly, our relationship came into being. Once he told me he had read about dissociation and realized that he had been "gone my whole life". He wanted to be real and spontaneous, but he could not imagine how that was possible if he were gone. He said I talked to him as if he were present and he was grateful for that.

In the second phase, he began to have many somatic symptoms. I will let you get a sense of his voice:

P: I have been psychically dead all my life. You told me dissociation was a type of death and I did not want to hear you, but now I agree.

A: You are having good insights, using your stress to come alive, and breaking your routines opens the possibility for more spontaneity.

P: It makes sense, but uh … first I thought the headaches were physical. I thought it was a tumor or cancer of some kind.
And I ache all over.

A: You are afraid of dying now that you are coming alive.

P: Yes, I have a red mark on my skin. I also fear I am going blind.
You know I am taking very seriously things I didn't take seriously before. The other day walking around my yard loving the flowers, I asked myself what kind of person am I? But I am being more spontaneous.
(Silent) Lots of bad stuff is coming up too. I used to say, it's just my unconscious.
(Silent) … but I can do a lot. It is me, and I can do something with what comes up … it is me.
I think about my psychic death, how I died and changed, not for the better.

Gradually over time, our relationship deepened. He began to bring me dreams and he began to grieve his past. He rarely cried, but he described crying at home. Always I was impressed how he would take these horrible feelings of pain and dread and say, "It must be good that I can feel this now".

He remembered a day when his father had demanded that he and the girls dig a basement under the house. This had been going on for months and his parents fought about it. The chimney actually began to tilt, so he said, due to their digging. The girls said they weren't going to dig anymore and their father went after them with a shovel. Dennis stepped in and got knocked to the ground while the girls ran away. Afterwards, he ran away too. He was given a ride to another part of town by his older brother. He said he was frightened. Then he accidentally saw his mother in front of the grocery store. He told me, *"And I felt my soul leave my body"*. When he returned home, he went to the edge of his garden, looking down on the neighboring houses and shouted, "Can't anyone see what is happening here? Help us! Help us!" No one came.

Another time when he told this story, he added:

> She saw me and had a goofy look on her face, was no help to me at all
> and that is when I had that experience; missing something. Thinking
> about my life ... and authenticity chipped away year after year and
> hardly anything left ... the effect they had on me emotionally ... and how
> I could not cover it up ... my friends must have seen it, but I do not think
> their souls left their bodies and they weren't being beaten and stuff.

In fact, previously Dennis had told me something was missing in him. He
didn't know what was missing, but he thought it had something to do with
not being real. I commented on how each time he told me his stories, they
were different. He was moved, saying his former analyst thought he was
obsessive, going over and over things again and again. He laughed, "Sounds
obsessive to me". I said it was sometimes difficult to notice little changes, that
sometimes he has a hint of a feeling in his words. He laughed and said, "Not
me".

Dennis came alive, and was able to describe mood changes within a single
day, something that surprised him. He always brought me dreams, having
learned they told him about himself. Then he told me of a day following one
of our sessions: he suddenly noticed that he no longer felt something was
missing in him: "I felt solid, like I have an inside. I walked around the house
saying, I am alive. I am alive". He began to play Elvis music on his recorder
and to dance.

Accompanied by himself now, he began to notice his dissociations. With
analysis, he began to observe what had happened just prior to them. More
and more he felt himself and in doing so, felt his need for contact with others.
He said, "It is hard to explain. I always knew what happened to me but now
when I think of it, I feel it. I feel lots of things now, not like before". He
deepened relationships and made new friends. He stayed in touch with his
siblings. He told me how much he valued his first analysts and that he loved
his partner. Much more could be said, but I am writing specifically about his
primal dissociations.

Discussion

Dissociation is a valuable ability. We all use it to help us focus and to facilitate our creativity. I believe differing forms of dissociation can be found in
each of the psychic positions—primal, paranoid schizoid, and depressive
(Eekhoff, 2022). In excess, primal dissociation takes the life out of the psyche
due to the extreme separation of body and mind. It interferes with the development of projective identification and an apparatus for thinking.

Receptivity seems an insufficient word to use in describing how I found
Dennis. If he was not transmitting truth via projective identification, but

rather maintaining stasis as a means of ridding himself of excess stimulation, how could I find him? If I mistakenly believed he was projectively identifying with me as a possible container for him, I might have been confused for a very long time. I would be mistaking my imaginings as coming from him. My illusion of at-one-ment with him would be my hallucination and delusion. Symbiotic at-one-ment in the hour must be of my experience of the two of us in whatever primal place we are. It enables growth in both participants.

Dennis was good at self-observation which he reported to me. He was not so good at self-reflection. His observations allowed me to reflect on our process and slowly over time to report it. This could be risky, as I had to constantly guard against providing more material for mimicry. Analysts since Freud have known this: Bergstein (2019) quoting Freud, "when the patient runs out of associations … we intervene on our own; we fill in the hints, draw undeniable conclusions, and give explicit utterances to what the patient only touched on in his associations" (1933, p. 12). When Dennis ran out of associations, which was frequent, he often simultaneously lost contact with me as a separate other. I became a symbolic equation at best. Our contact was proximal, only at a physical concrete level. At first, I thought this was his distancing from me, but I came to understand in that moment he was lost to himself. He was dissociating body from mind, and lost contact with himself, having no sensorial awareness. Differentiation of himself from me too was lost.

Since often these patients are so concrete as to be unable to associate, the filling in happens unconsciously first at the level of bodily relations (Bleger, 1967). Even when the patient and the analyst are speaking to each other, it is the sound and rhythm of the speech that is of primary importance. There is not aggression or defense since the union forecloses an awareness of twoness. The interaction merely is concrete, material, true in a physical manner. Any elaboration by the analyst is not possible under those circumstances, because as I reported earlier, the patient will say, "I didn't say that". Such a concrete comment is evidence of a difficulty in thinking and learning from experience (Bion, 1962a, 1962b). As Goldberg (2021) says, "where there is dissociation, the function of association is disabled. This means that the therapeutic function of receptivity and introjective identification are much reduced in the treatment of dissociation" (p. 125).

Conclusion

Using a clinical case, I have described somato-psychic dissociative states that foreclose meaning-making rather than use the sensual to find meaning. Such states, when shared in the analytic hour, can be transformed so that experience is not only observable but can be reflected upon and used for the coherence and development of the self. Learning from experience is then possible.

I have described a kind of analytic reverie that includes physical proximity, sensation, and sound, and rhythm and synchronicity. I have used Bleger's

(1967) description of this as symbiotic. Being receptive of primal states of mind requires the perception of bodily experience. These states are always nonverbal, and in fact may never be fully symbolized in language. Receptivity via a body relation also requires the analyst be present and attuned not to the symbolic order but to the perceptual order of immediate experience. Perceptual identity of both patient and analyst enables growth. Analytic receptivity enables previously unrepresented and poorly represented states to move from presentations of experience to representations of experience.

References

Alvarez, A. (1992). *Live company.* Routledge.

Bergstein, A. (2019). *Bion and Meltzer's expeditions into unmapped mental life, beyond the spectrum in psychoanalysis.* Routledge.

Bion, W.R. (1958). On arrogance. *International Journal of Psycho-Analysis*, 39, 144–146.

Bion, W.R. (1962a). A psycho-analytic theory of thinking. *International Journal of Psycho-Analysis*, 43, 306–310. [Reprinted as "A theory of thinking", in W.R. Bion, *Second thoughts.* Karnac, 1984 (pp. 110–119).]

Bion, W.R. (1962b). *Learning from experience.* Heinemann. [Reprinted Karnac, 1984.]

Bion, W.R. (1965). *Transformations.* Heinemann. [Reprinted Karnac, 1984.]

Bion, W.R. (1967). *Wilford Bion: Los Angeles seminars and supervision*, Ed. J. Aguayo & B. Malin (2013). Routledge.

Bion, W.R. (1970). *Attention and interpretation.* Tavistock. [Reprinted Karnac, 1984.]

Bion, W.R. (1992). *Cogitations.* New extended edition. Karnac.

Bleger, J. (1967). *Symbiosis and ambiguity: A psychoanalytic study*, Ed. J. Churcher & L. Bleger, Trans. S. Rogers, L. Bleger, & J. Churcher (2013). Routledge.

Bollas, C. (1987). *The shadow of the object: Psychoanalysis of the unthought known.* Free Association Books.

Civitarese, G. (2012). *The violence of emotions: Bion and post-Bionian psychoanalysis.* Routledge.

Civitarese, G. (2015). Transformations in hallucinosis and the receptivity of the analyst. *International Journal of Psycho-Analysis*, 96, 1091–1116.

Eekhoff, J.K. (2019). *Trauma and primitive mental states: An object relations perspective.* Routledge.

Eekhoff, J.K. (2022). *Bion and primitive mental states: Trauma and the symbiotic link.* Routledge.

Ferenczi, S. (1929). The unwelcome child and his death-instinct. *International Journal of Psycho-Analysis*, 10, 125–129. [Reprinted in *Final contributions to the problems and methods of psycho-analysis* (pp. 102–107), Karnac, 1994.]

Ferenczi, S. (1933). Confusion of the tongues between the adults and the child—(The language of tenderness and of passion). In *Final contributions to the problems and methods of psycho-analysis* (1994, pp. 156–167). Karnac.

Ferenczi, S. (1955). Notes and fragments. In *Final contributions to the problems and methods of psycho-analysis* (pp. 216–279). Karnac. [Reprinted Karnac, 1994.]

Freud, S. (1933). Revision of the theory of dreams. In *S.E.* (Vol. 22, pp. 7–30). Hogarth.

Goldberg, P. (2021). Embodiment, dissociation, and the rhythm of life. In C. Harrang, D. Tillotson, & N.C. Winters (Eds.), *Body as psychoanalytic object: Clinical applications from Winnicott to Bion and beyond* (pp. 118–133). Routledge.

Lombardi, R. (2017). *Body-mind dissociation in psychoanalysis: Development after Bion*. Routledge.

Meltzer, D. (1986). *Studies in extended metapsychology: Clinical applications of Bion's ideas*. Clunie Press.

Mitrani, J.L. (2001). *Ordinary people and extra-ordinary protections*. New Library of Psychoanalysis. Brunner-Routledge.

Monteiro, J.S. (2023). *Bion's theory of dreams: A visionary model of the mind*. Routledge.

Skogstad, W. (2013). Impervious and intrusive: The impenetrable object in transference and countertransference. *International Journal of Psychoanalysis*, 94, 221–238.

Index